Frozen Section Library

Series Editor
Philip T. Cagle, MD
Houston, Texas, USA

For other titles published in this series, go to
http://www.springer.com/series/7869

Frozen Section Library: Bone

Omar Hameed, MBChB

University of Alabama at Birmingham, AL, USA

Shi Wei, MD, PhD

University of Alabama at Birmingham, AL, USA

Gene P. Siegal, MD, PhD

University of Alabama at Birmingham, AL, USA

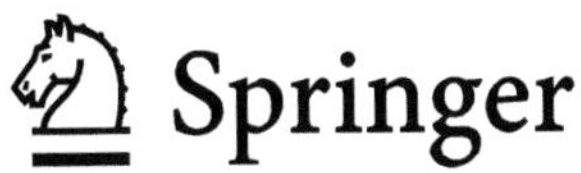

Springer

Omar Hameed, MBChB
Associate Professor of Pathology and Surgery
Department of Pathology
University of Alabama at Birmingham
Birmingham, AL, USA
ohameed@uab.edu

Shi Wei, MD, PhD
Assistant Professor
Department of Pathology
University of Alabama at Birmingham
Birmingham, AL, USA
swei@uab.edu

Gene P. Siegal, MD, PhD
R. W. Mowry Endowed Professor of Pathology
Director, Division of Anatomic Pathology
Executive Vice-Chair – Pathology, UAB Health System
Department of Pathology
University of Alabama at Birmingham
Birmingham, AL, USA
gsiegal@uab.edu

ISSN 1868-4157   e-ISSN 1868-4165
ISBN 978-1-4419-8375-6   ISBN 978-1-4419-8376-3 (eBook)
DOI 10.1007/978-1-4419-8376-3
Springer New York Dordrecht Heidelberg London

Library of Congress Control Number: 2011921258

Springer is part of Springer Science+Business Media (www.springer.com)

To my parents, my dearest wife, Chura, and my daughters,
Shilan and Sara

OH

To my loving wife, Mei, for her unending support,
and my wonderful children, Johnny and Erica

SW

To all those who have taught me...my mentors,
my trainees and most assuredly my family
- from Sandy to Marley and all those in between.

GPS

Series Preface

For over 100 years, the frozen section has been utilized as a tool for the rapid diagnosis of specimens while a patient is undergoing surgery, usually under general anesthesia, as a basis for making immediate treatment decisions. Frozen section diagnosis is often a challenge for the pathologist who must render a diagnosis that has crucial import for the patient in a minimal amount of time. In addition to the need for rapid recall of differential diagnoses, there are many pitfalls and artifacts that add to the risk of frozen section diagnosis that are not present with permanent sections of fully processed tissues that can be examined in a more leisurely fashion. Despite the century-long utilization of frozen sections, most standard pathology textbooks, both general and subspecialty, largely ignore the topic of frozen sections. Few textbooks have ever focused exclusively on frozen section diagnosis and those textbooks that have done so are now out-of-date and have limited illustrations.

The Frozen Section Library Series is meant to provide convenient, user-friendly handbooks for each organ system to expedite use in the rushed frozen section situation. These books are small and lightweight, copiously color illustrated with images of actual frozen sections, highlighting pitfalls, artifacts, and differential diagnosis. The advantages of a series of organ-specific handbooks, in addition to the ease-of-use and manageable size, are that (1) a series allows more comprehensive coverage of more diagnoses, both common and rare, than a single volume that tries to highlight a limited number of diagnoses for each organ and (2) a series allows more detailed insight by permitting experienced authorities to emphasize the peculiarities of frozen section for each organ system.

As a handbook for practicing pathologists, these books will be indispensable aids to diagnosis and avoiding dangers in one of the most challenging situations that pathologists encounter. Rapid consideration of differential diagnoses and how to avoid traps caused by frozen section artifacts are emphasized in these handbooks. A series of concise, easy-to-use, well-illustrated handbooks alleviates the often frustrating and time-consuming, sometimes futile, process of searching through bulky textbooks that are unlikely to illustrate or discuss pathologic diagnoses from the perspective of frozen sections in the first place. Tables and charts will provide guidance for differential diagnosis of various histologic patterns. Touch preparations, which are used for some organs such as central nervous system or thyroid more often than others, are appropriately emphasized and illustrated according to the need for each specific organ.

This series is meant to benefit practicing surgical pathologists, both community and academic, and to pathology residents and fellows; and also to provide valuable perspectives to surgeons, surgery residents, and fellows who must rely on frozen section diagnosis by their pathologists. Most of all, we hope that this series contributes to the improved care of patients who rely on the frozen section to help guide their treatment.

Philip T. Cagle, MD

Preface

This monograph attempts to provide for the trainee, as well as the seasoned pathologist with limited exposure to bone lesions, an introduction to the most common forms of tumor and tumor-like conditions of bone seen in North American clinical practice. We have purposely avoided demonstrating exotica which few, if any of us, would hope to see in a lifetime of experience even in an academic medical center. For example, we have purposely avoided demonstrating examples of primary smooth and striated muscle tumors of bone; likewise the lipogenic tumors and neural tumors of bone have not been reported. Rather, we have focused, in eight chapters, on the common cartilaginous and osteogenic tumors, fibrogenic tumors, small cell tumors, giant cell tumors, epithelial tumors, and vascular tumors. We have also highlighted, where appropriate, reactive, cystic, and reparative conditions that are often mistaken for primary neoplasms in their presentation and have further supplemented the actual frozen section in many cases with representative radiographic images to help the pathologist in understanding the breadth and depth of such lesions. Furthermore, although a particular interest of ours, we have avoided discussing the cytogenetic and molecular genetic characteristics of many of the demonstrated lesions as well as avoided the ultrastructural and immunophenotypic characteristics, leaving these for the primary literature or the many outstanding themed textbooks in the field which we have selectively highlighted at the end of this monograph. In an attempt to be consistent with the other books in this series, we have tried to minimize the text and rather provided full color images of the histopathology, often at different magnifications, to the help serve as an atlas for those confronted with an unknown lesion. Lastly, rather than attempting to take photomicrographs of the most idealized fields in a tumor or tumor-like condition, we have purposely tried to mix such images with those that are less than ideal to give the reader a sense of the challenges faced in the actual practice of frozen section interpretation of such lesions. We hope you benefit from this approach and benefit from this treatise.

Birmingham, 2011

Omar Hameed
Shi Wei
Gene P. Siegal

Contents

Chapter 1
Introduction

Orthopedic Pathology, specifically tumors of bone and related conditions, has a reputation as a diagnostically difficult area of practice. The reasons for this are multiple and probably include the reality that such lesions are quite rare (representing <1% of all cases seen in typical community practices) so the "average" pathologist may have limited experience in dealing with such cases and may not develop a sense of confidence in recognizing these lesions. The second cause is the realization that bone has only a limited number of ways to respond to an insult and thus many lesions overlap morphologically at the gross, microscopic, and ultrastructural levels. Thirdly, pathologists have developed a keen insight into what to expect histologically when observing the gross features of a pathologic condition. In bone, the radiograph or special radiographic study (MRI, CT scan, bone scan, and PET scan) acts invariablely as the "gross pathology." Pathologists, although highly trained, have minimal exposure to radiologic practice and might be helpless in interpreting the images themselves, and with lack of immediate access to musculoskeletal radiologists, usually do not know what the "gross pathology" looks like. This series of challenges is heightened by the isolation of the frozen section suite in many North American hospitals. One further cause for the uncomfortable state many pathologists find themselves in when having to deal with lesions of bone is the incorrect notion that such tumors are by their nature invariably "bone hard" and thus not susceptible to interpretation by frozen section analysis. Nothing could be further from the truth; virtually all lesions of bone including those that are "bone producing" have tissue soft enough to cut on a cryostat, as has been demonstrated for more than 100 years at

1

O. Hameed et al., *Frozen Section Library: Bone*, Frozen Section Library,
DOI 10.1007/978-1-4419-8376-3_1, © Springer Science+Business Media, LLC 2011

the Mayo Clinic (which has perhaps the largest collection of bone tumors in the world). Thus, diagnoses obtained by intraoperative consultation, i.e., by frozen sections, are readily possible.

We remain at a point in time, more than half a century since Jaffe defined the so-called triad for the diagnosis of tumors of bone, where a partnership still is required between the clinician who has knowledge of the demographic and clinical features of the patient presenting to him, the radiologist with his ever expanding armamentarium of techniques and instruments, and the pathologist who bring his unique skill set to reach the proper diagnosis. This becomes even more critical in the high-pressure environment of the frozen section room. It is requisite that this triad of cooperation be in place either before the operation begins or depending on the emergent nature of the presentation, during the operation. One would be severely remiss, if one failed to personally review the radiographic images and/or radiology reports or, if not possible, to ask the clinician or radiologist what the appropriately radiographic images revealed. Although it seems easy and simple to say, we find often in our consultation practice failure to follow this most simple of rules. Such failure invariably leads the pathologist down a pathway from which he or she cannot easily recover; so for example, without the knowledge of the patient's demographics, it might result in the pathologist pontificating that in this 65-year-old patient with a small blue round cell tumor that neuroblastoma is a reasonable choice in the differential diagnosis. Similarly, a pure cartilaginous lesion in the phalange of a 12-year old is probably not going to be a chondrosarcoma. Giant cell tumor of bone, giant cell reparative granuloma, and so-called brown tumor of hyperthyroidism often have extensive overlapping histopathologic features and is it only by knowing the patient's age, gender, presentation, clinical and laboratory studies, and radiographic appearances can one hope to reach a reasonable and appropriate diagnosis. More subtle, if one has a lesion that appears to be benign fibrous histiocytoma, one best be sure it is not, in fact, really a case of metaphyseal fibrous defect/non-ossifying fibroma that was in inadvertently biopsied as the histology is essentially identical.

By following the standard rules of good practice as defined by Jaffe, it should be relatively easy to reach a very narrow differential diagnosis or the one "correct" diagnosis on the frozen section biopsy interpretation; however, it is also important to realize that sometimes it is not wise or even possible to do so and here the experience of the pathologist is critical in being able to share his or her uncertainty honestly with the surgeon. It goes without saying that calling a benign osseous lesion an osteosarcoma is not acceptable and could lead to rapid consequences from which one could not recover. Thus, whenever there is even a reasonable doubt, it is often best to say you favor such and such but need to do further analysis or more definitive studies and the final diagnosis will be deferred. Lastly, often times the surgeon does not really need or want the final diagnosis but really wants to know whether there is sufficient material to reach that diagnosis in a one-step operation. Here again experience and judgment are critical so if, for example, one is suspecting primary lymphoma of bone, one will need to perform flow cytometry, perhaps touch preps and molecular diagnostics, and one cannot reasonably do that on a limited sample provided for frozen sectioning. One would hopefully be perfectly comfortable in saying that there is a high degree of suspicion for lymphoma or a malignant lymhoreticular process, but that additional tissues are requested for special studies.

In this treatise, we follow a simple decision tree which has as its center six key questions:

1. What are the key demographic features (age, sex, and race) of the patient and does the patient have a relevant past history (previous cancer diagnosis, genetic disease, radiation history, etc.) or altered laboratory values?
2. What do the radiographic images show and what is the radiologic differential diagnosis?
3. Which bone or bones are involved and where in the bone (surface, cortex, or intramedullary)?
4. Is it a long bone or flat bone and if the former is it epiphyseal, diaphyseal, or metaphyseal in location?
5. Is it solid or cystic (or both); what are the main features of the lesion and is it producing a particular extracellular matrix (e.g., osteoid, chondroid, or myxoid); and what are the principal cell types involved (e.g., small cells, giant cells, and epithelial cells)?
6. Do the clinical data, radiologic findings and histopathologic features come together into a logical picture?

Sure it is possible that you are seeing in the frozen section room the first reported case of a chordoma in the metatarsal of a teenager but really how reasonable a diagnosis is that? By following this strategy, we believe that one stays out of trouble, can create a reasonable differential diagnosis and will not be operating on luck. Indeed you will be engaged in the best of good practice.

Chapter 2
Bone/Osteoid Producing Lesions

There are many lesions that are associated with reactive new bone formation; this chapter predominantly covers those in which deposition of osteoid/bone matrix represents the primary pathological process. The key in recognizing these lesions is the identification of osteoid or woven bone (vs. lamellar bone) on the frozen section slide. Osteoid is the organic nonmineralized matrix of bone and, being predominantly composed of type I collagen fibers, appears homogeneously eosinophilic and almost keloid-like in nature. This matrix is almost always associated with osteoblasts within clear spaces or halos. Bone matrix is further classified as lamellar or woven depending upon the predominant fiber arrangement of its collagen. In lamellar bone, the bone collagen fibers are arranged in tightly packed stacks that are parallel to one another but run at slightly different angles so that the bone appears to be layered. Moreover, the osteoblasts/osteocytes within lamellar bone also run parallel to the collagen fibers. After about 3 years of age, normal compact (cortical) and cancellous (trabecular, spongy, and medullary) bone exclusively consist of lamellar bone. In contrast, woven bone is found in the fetal skeleton, in the growing parts of the skeleton in infants and adolescents, and in processes in which there is very rapid bone production secondary to neoplastic or nonneoplastic conditions. Accordingly, identification of lesional woven bone and its distinction from adjacent lamellar bone is crucial during frozen section evaluation. This is based on the fact that, in contrast to lamellar bone, woven bone is characterized by the random distribution of its collagen fibers and the irregular distribution of osteoblasts within it. Although the distinction between

O. Hameed et al., *Frozen Section Library: Bone*, Frozen Section Library,
DOI 10.1007/978-1-4419-8376-3_2, © Springer Science+Business Media, LLC 2011

lamellar and woven bone can, for the most part, be made using regular bright-field microscopy, the process can be facilitated with the use of polarized light.

Once the presence of bone matrix has been established, one has to determine if its presence is primary or secondary in nature, a determination often compounded by the fact that many frozen section samples include intermixed curettings from the lamellar bone immediately adjacent to the lesion in question. In most cases, where the production of new bone is secondary, its presence tends to be focal in nature and closely intermixed with other reactive elements including hemorrhage and osteoclast giant cells. Moreover, there is usually a zonal distribution which may not be easily appreciated in curetting specimens. On the other hand, bone production in most cases of primary bone-producing lesions tends to more extensive and generally not intimately associated with reactive elements, that, if present, also tend to be peripherally located.

As stated throughout this book, evaluation of any bone lesion (intraoperatively or otherwise) should not be made independently from the clinical (age of the patient, bone involved, and portion of bone involved) and radiological findings. This is no less true for the bone-producing lesions discussed in this chapter, which, although having overlapping histological features, can have quite distinct clinical and/or radiological features that are crucial to arriving at the correct diagnosis.

FRACTURE CALLUS

Although fractures are numerically one of the most frequent bone "disorders," intraoperative consultation is infrequently requested unless the fracture is thought to be pathological in nature. Although acute fractures can be hemorrhagic and display some fragmented bone trabeculae, these changes are nonspecific and are very difficult to evaluate in the setting of the artifacts associated with frozen sections. Subacute fractures (meaning a few days old, rather than hours or weeks) may also display empty osteocyte lacunae and necrosis of marrow. Older fractures that do not readily heal and, as noted above, those that are thought to be pathologic, are more frequently sampled to rule out the presence of an occult neoplasm or infection. In the absence of these etiologies mimicking the natural healing process that moves from fibrosis to chondrogenesis to osteogenesis in long bones, one observes irregular islands and trabeculae of osteoid with an intervening, variably cellular reactive spindle-cell stroma. Scattered osteoclasts are frequently present (Figs. 2.1 and 2.2) as are islands of cartilage (Fig. 2.3). It is very important to know that there is a history of trauma, otherwise

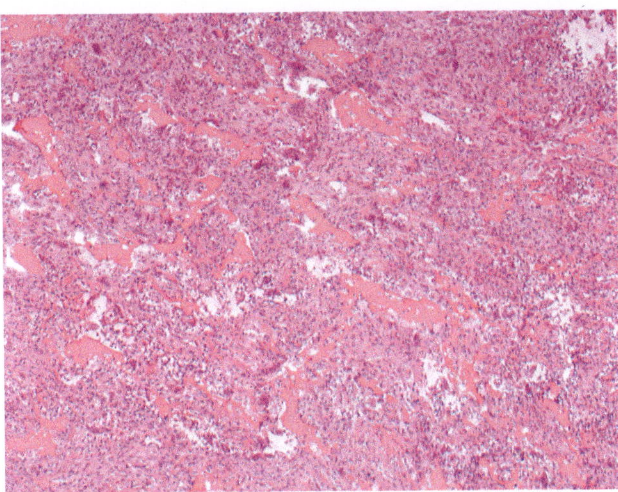

FIGURE 2.1 Low power view of a fracture callus showing a cellular infiltrate in which scattered eosinophilic islands of osteoid are evident.

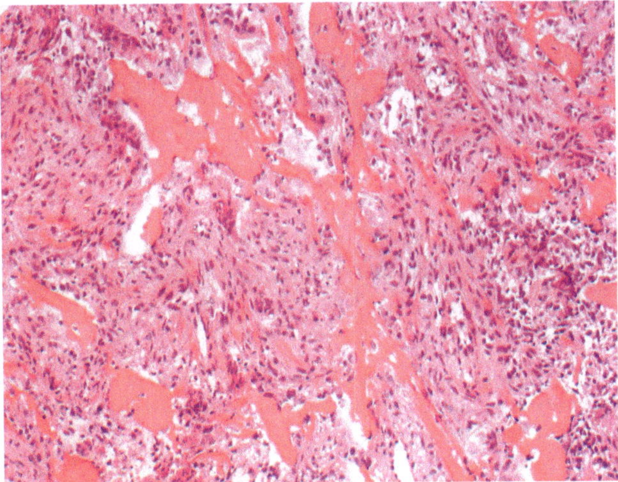

FIGURE 2.2 On higher magnification, this fracture callus shows a predominantly spindle-cell component in which scattered osteoclasts are evident. Notice that although the osteoid islands are mostly irregular in shape, one starts to appreciate the somewhat parallel alignment of these islands (running downwards and to the right in this field). Such an appearance is strongly in favor of reactive, nonneoplastic osteoid deposition.

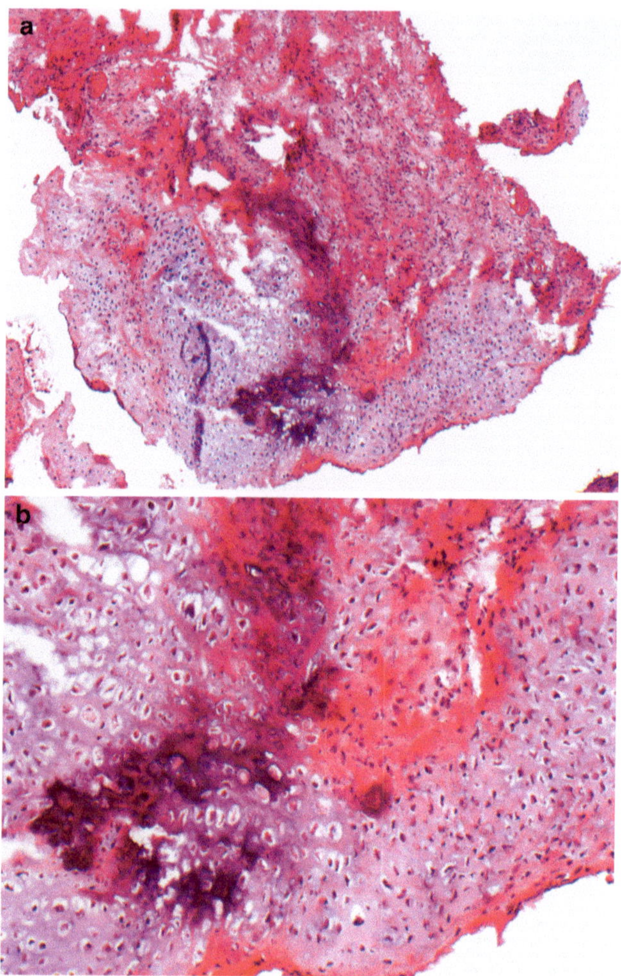

FIGURE 2.3 Hyaline cartilage is frequently a component of fracture callus (**a**). The presence of orderly endochondral ossification (**b**) is another helpful feature of benignity.

one might misinterpret the osteoid as being neoplastic in nature. Of note, primary bone-producing neoplasms are rarely the sites of fracture unless radiographically evident and quite large.

There are a few histological parameters that help to distinguish bone (and cartilage) formation by tumor from that secondary to trauma; however, it might be difficult to appreciate them in frozen sections. Although reactive osteoid may start off focally lacelike in appearance (Fig. 2.4), it rapidly acquires a microtrabecular to trabecular architecture as it matures, and there is almost always a zonation of orderly maturation (Fig. 2.5).

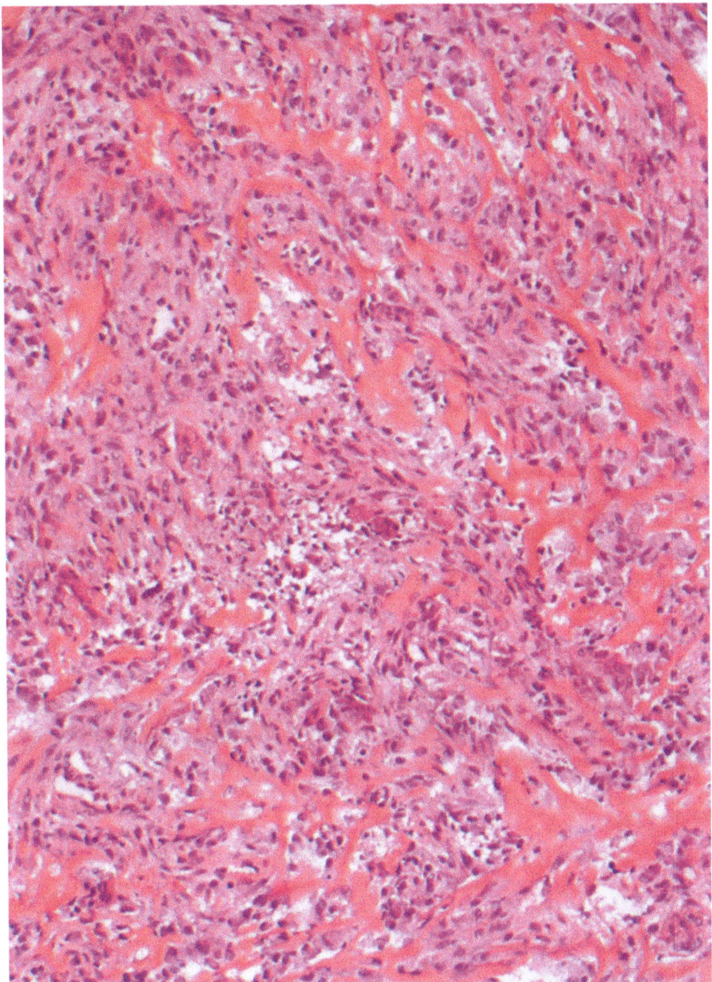

FIGURE 2.4 The presence of focal lace-like areas of osteoid deposition in a fracture callus can be worrisome for neoplasia. However, this focus also displays an edematous spindle-cell stroma with scattered inflammatory cells and osteoclasts and no evidence of cytological atypia.

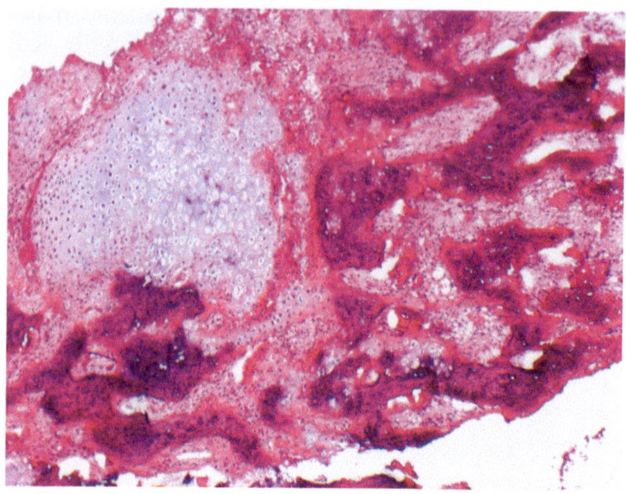

FIGURE 2.5 With time, there is progressively more bone deposition in a fracture callus and the orderly trabecular pattern of deposition is one of the best clues to suggest a nonneoplastic process.

In contrast, neoplastic osteoid invariably has a lace-like or sheet-like appearance (see below) and there is no orderly maturation.

REACTIVE BONE

In addition to being a component of fracture callus, as noted earlier, reactive bone may be seen accompanying a variety of bone infections with secondary attempts at healing/repair. As such, this often surrounds the lesion in question or is part of an accompanying reactive periosteal new bone formation. The orderly parallel arrangement of the trabeculae/microtrabeculae in reactive bone (Fig. 2.6) is characteristic.

OSTEOMA

The characteristic clinical and radiographic findings of this benign lesion, when linked to its classic location in the skull and sinuses, make it an unlikely frozen section sample. Moreover, its dense bony nature would make sectioning virtually impossible.

OSTEOID OSTEOMA

This bone-forming tumor is relatively common, representing at least 10% of all benign bone neoplasms. Most patients are between 10 and 30 years of age and the lesion most frequently involves the cortex of long bones. One of osteoid osteoma's characteristic

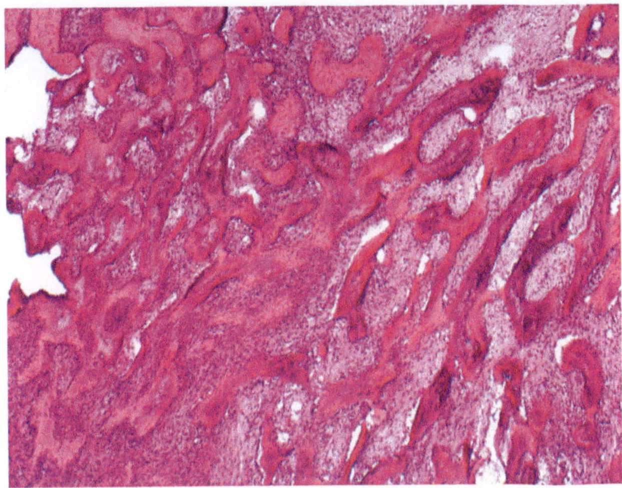

FIGURE 2.6   The pattern of bone deposition in reactive bone is very similar to that seen in fracture callus.

symptoms is progressive pain, easily relieved by ingestion of nonsteroidal anti-inflammatory drugs. Radiologically, a radiolucent "nidus" surrounded by sclerotic bone is quite characteristic (Fig. 2.7). Histologically, the nidus is composed of vascularized fibroconnective tissue in which osteoid or mineralized new bone is evident. This new bone is usually arranged in microtrabecular arrays, lined by plump appositional osteoblasts, and surrounded by sclerotic bone. Given its characteristic clinical and radiological features, osteoid osteoma is rarely sampled intraoperatively. Moreover, definitive treatment by radiofrequency ablation or cryotherapy is not infrequently performed prior to pathological confirmation of the diagnosis. Unfortunately, in most of these cases, one sees only markedly fragmented nonviable bone (sometimes referred to as "bone dust") that is nondiagnostic histologically.

OSTEOBLASTOMA

The histological features of this neoplasm are identical to those of osteoid osteoma except for the fact that it has an expanded growth potential. It also arises in adolescence and young adulthood and frequently involves the cortices of long bones; however, spinal vertebrae are also a common site of involvement (Fig. 2.8). As noted above, microtrabecular arrays of osteoid or woven bone lined by plump osteoblasts dominate the histological appearance (Fig. 2.9). Some cases can be significantly more cellular being composed of

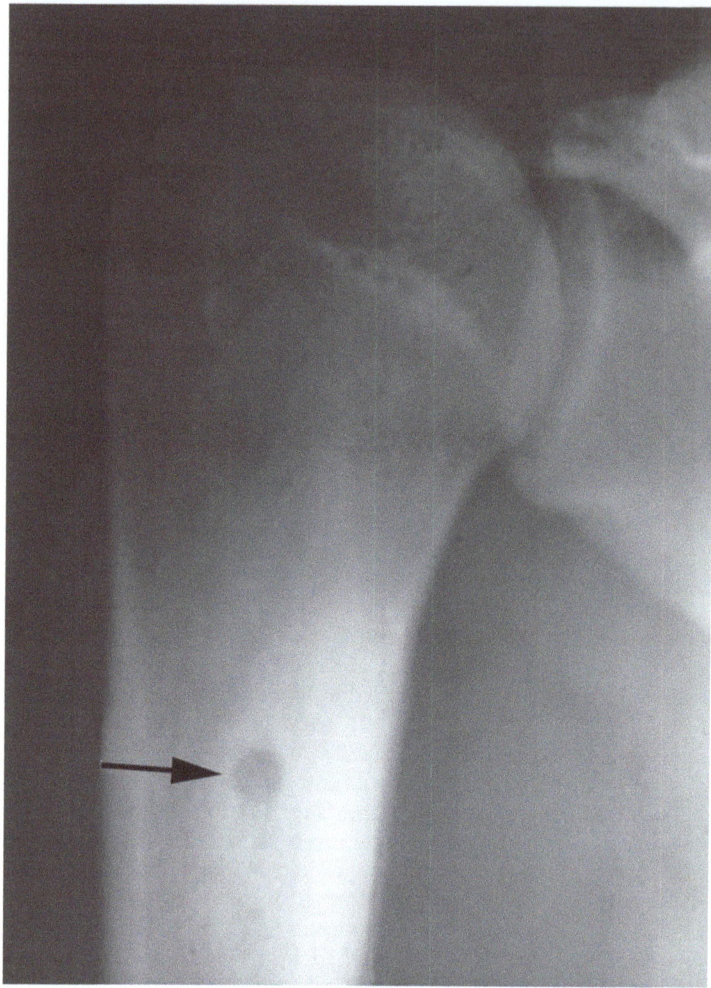

FIGURE 2.7 An osteoid osteoma of the humerus showing the characteristic lucent nidus (*arrow*) surrounded by sclerotic bone.

FIGURE 2.8 An osteoblastoma appearing on plain radiograph (**a**) as an expansile lesion in the transverse process of the third lumbar vertebra (*arrows*). The expansile nature of the lesion is also quite apparent on the CT scan (**b**) (images courtesy of Dr. Michael J. Klein, Hospital for Special Surgery, New York, NY).

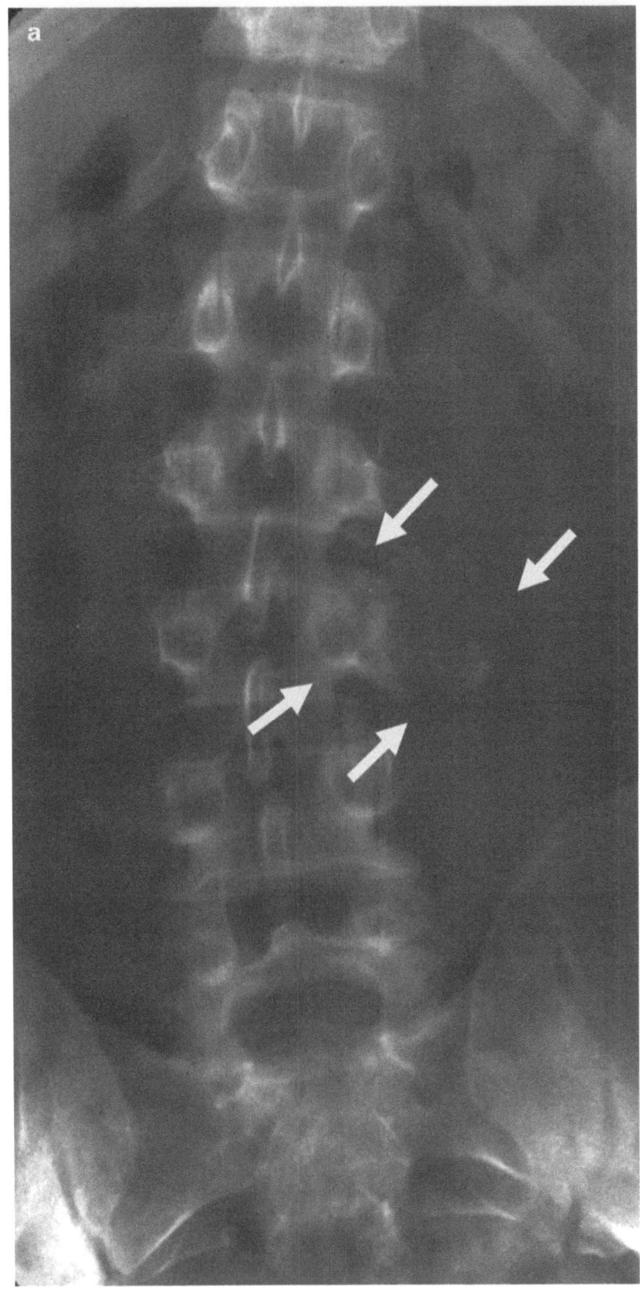

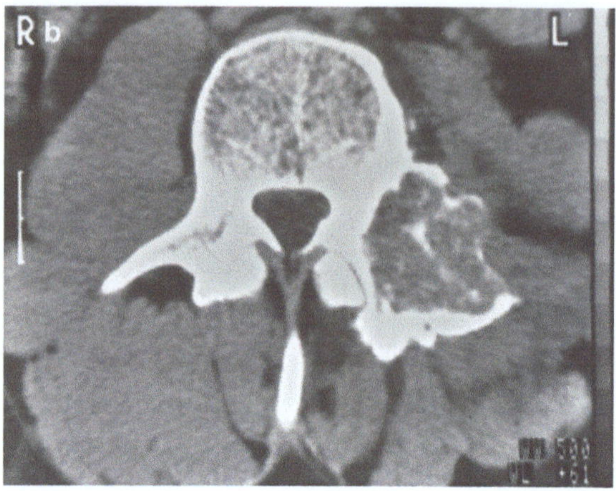

Figure 2.8 (continued)

sheets of tumor cells with less easily discernable osteoid (Fig. 2.10). Lack of nuclear pleomorphism in the conventional forms of this neoplasm is one feature that is useful to distinguish them from other variants including the "aggressive" and "epithelioid" types. Pathologists need to be aware that there is a histologic continuum between conventional osteoblastoma and osteosarcoma, with the osteoblastoma variants in the middle. Considering the histological (and radiological) difficulty in recognizing these variants and distinguishing them from osteosarcoma, it is prudent to defer the diagnosis of atypical cases to permanent sections.

OSTEOSARCOMA

Excluding hematopoietic tumors, osteosarcoma is the most common primary malignant neoplasm of bone. The peak incidence is late childhood and adolescence, but there is another peak in patients over 50 years where most cases develop secondarily in preexisting bone lesions, such as Paget's disease or following irradiation. The metaphyses of long bones (femur, tibia, and humerus) are the most common sites of involvement, isolated diaphysial involvement is rare, while involvement of the epiphyses of long bones or small bones of the hands and feet is exceptionally uncommon. The tumor may also involve the jaws, skull and axial skeleton. A significant proportion of patients presents with pain (often dull and unremitting) with or without a palpable mass. Radiologically, there is almost always evidence of a destructive bony lesion, often with evidence of new bone formation. There may also be an interrupted periosteal reaction (Fig. 2.11).

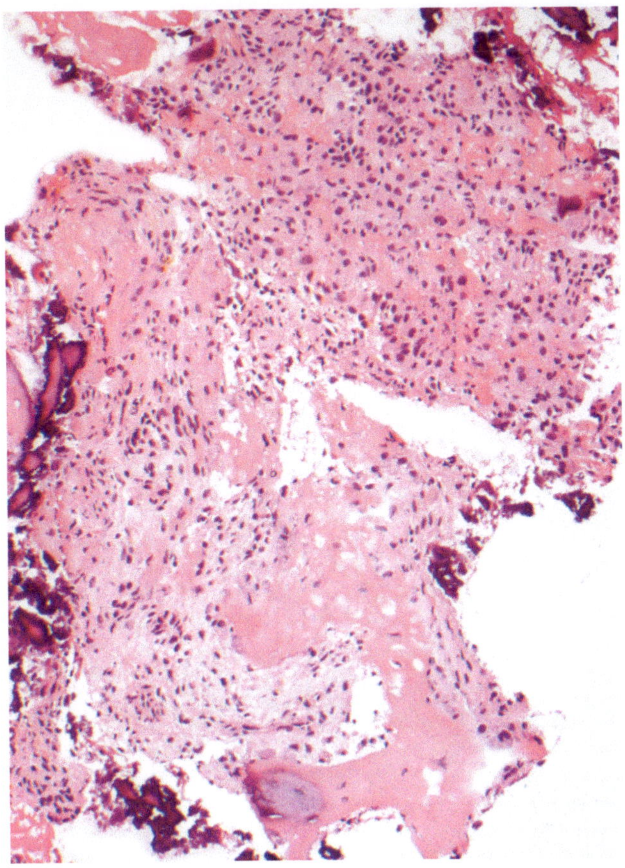

FIGURE 2.9 Although not very cellular, one can appreciate a somewhat monotonous cell population in this osteoblastoma. The faintly staining microtrabecular osteoid in the upper right portion of the image is surrounded by appositional osteoblasts.

The histological hallmark of osteosarcoma is the presence of tumor osteoid or bone being formed directly by tumor cells. Similar to that seen in fracture callus and osteoblastoma, tumor osteoid has unique tinctorial properties on hematoxylin and eosin-stained sections appearing as dense, pink, amorphous material that is often described as "hard." As noted above, osteoid may have a lace-like (Fig. 2.12) or sheet-like (Fig. 2.13) appearance in osteosarcomas. Although subclassification of osteosarcomas as osteoblastic, chondroblastic, or fibroblastic based upon the predominant matrix produced has no prognostic impact, identification of a significant

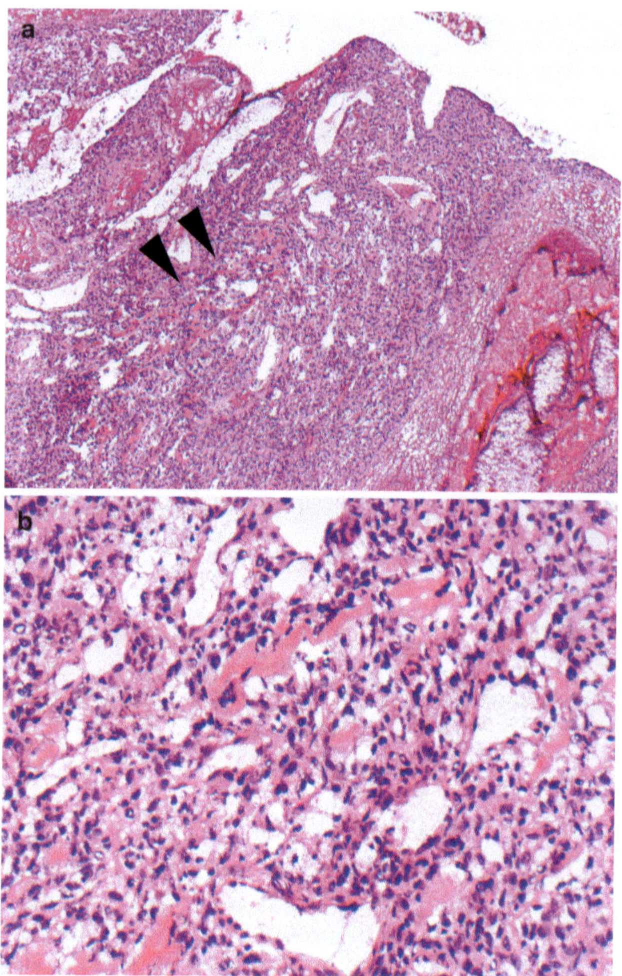

FIGURE 2.10 This osteoblastoma was markedly cellular (**a**) to the extent that osteoid could only be focally identified (*arrowheads*). Higher magnification (**b**) confirms the hypercellular nature of the neoplasm and better displays the osteoid matrix. One should always remember that nuclear atypia is exaggerated on frozen sections and thus be careful not to make a diagnosis of osteosarcoma based solely on that feature.

chondroid or spindle-cell component *independent of* the osteoid matrix may also be a useful clue toward the diagnosis. The neoplastic tumor cells are usually seen intermixed within the osteoid matrix but occasionally may appear to be in direct opposition to it; they may even be condensed around it in a palisaded fashion

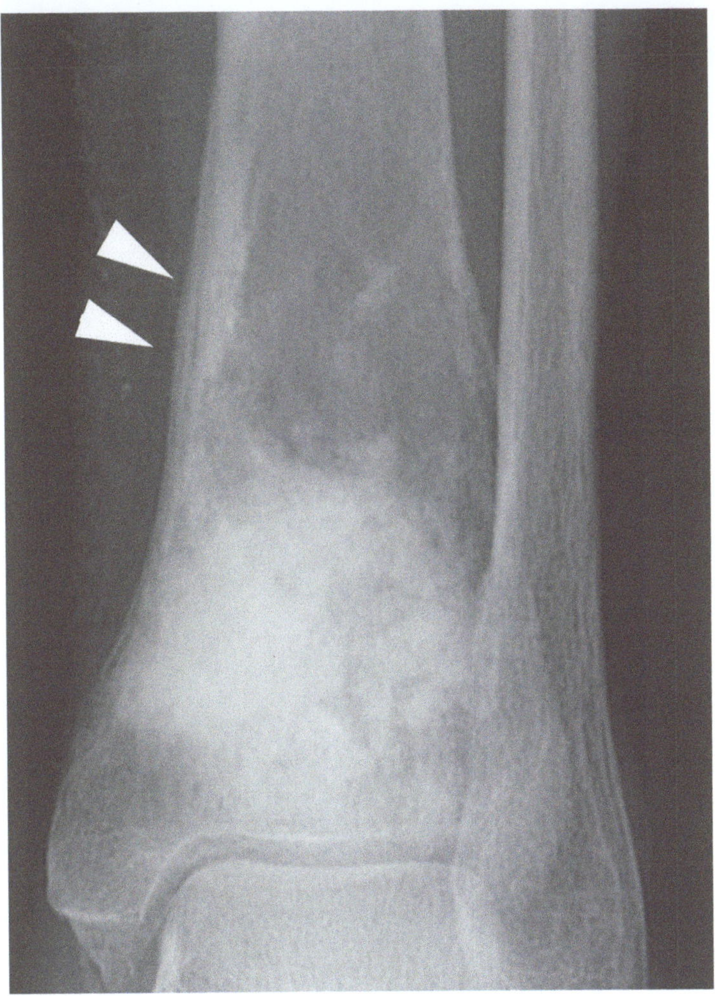

FIGURE 2.11 An osteosarcoma of the lower tibia that is predominantly osteoblastic and also shows lucent areas. Notice the irregular cortex and slightly lifted periosteum (*arrowheads*).

(Fig. 2.13). Morphologically, the tumor cells are usually round to polyhedral in shape and significant pleomorphism is usually present (Figs. 2.12 and 2.14). In other cases, the tumor cells can have a predominantly spindle-cell morphology (Fig. 2.15). It is important to note, however, that significant nuclear atypia may not always be present in conventional high-grade lesions, in that case

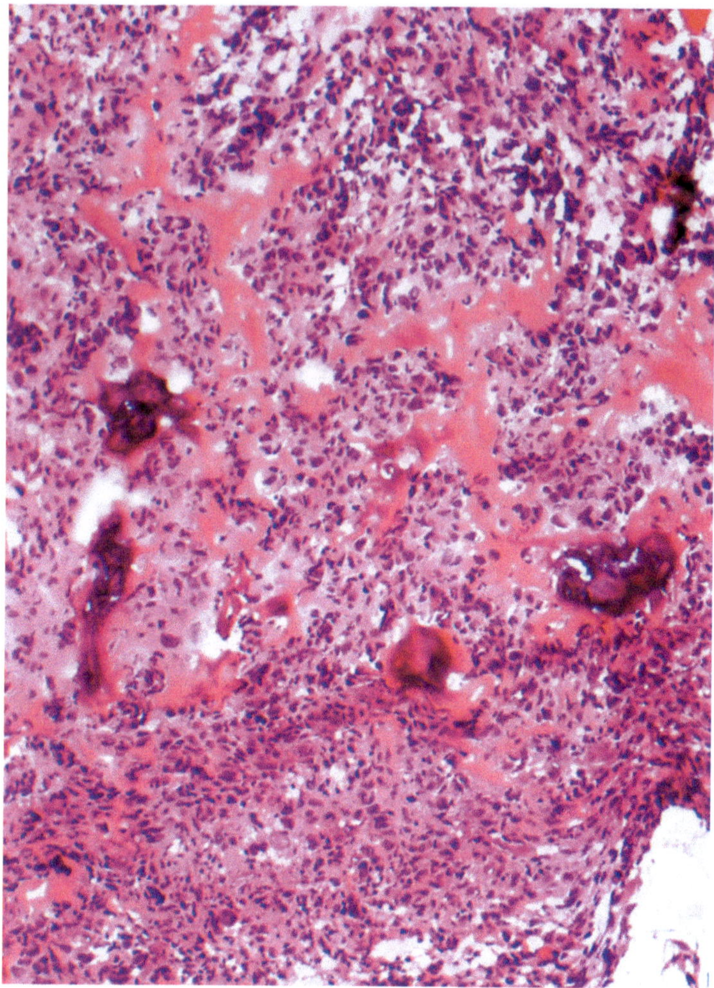

FIGURE 2.12 A typical appearance of osteosarcoma on frozen section where one sees a very cellular lesion with characteristic irregular lace-like osteoid deposition. Notice to the hyperchromatic nature of the tumor cells.

the radiological evidence of a destructive bony lesion can be one of the most useful clues to suggest the diagnosis of osteosarcoma.

In addition to *conventional intramedullary osteosarcoma*, the prototypical central osteosarcoma discussed above, there are other variants of osteosarcoma, including some that are potentially more challenging diagnostically.

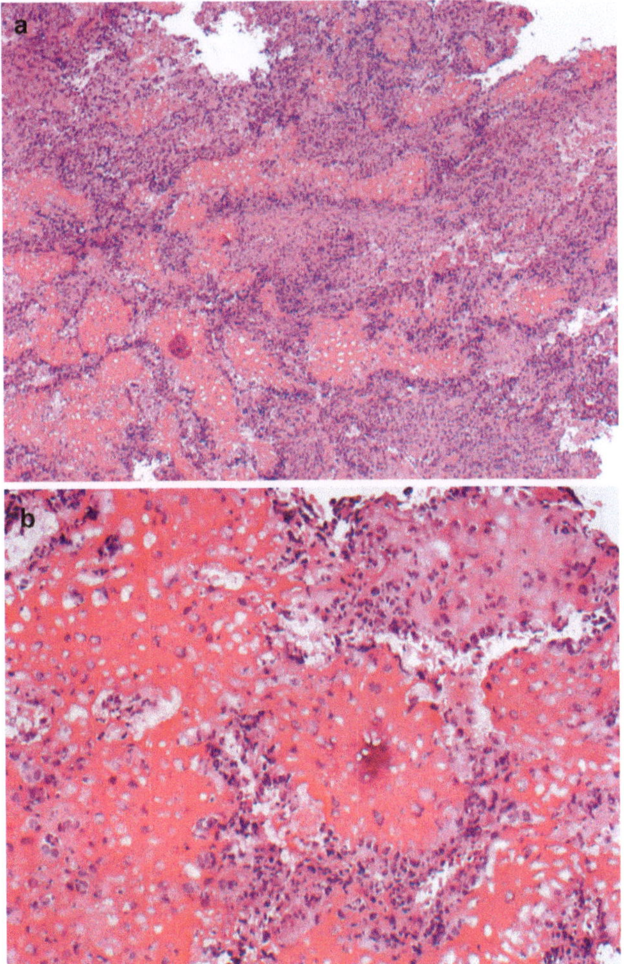

FIGURE 2.13 Another osteosarcoma in which the neoplastic osteoid had more of a sheet-like pattern of deposition (**a**). There is also prominent palisading of tumor cells around the osteoid matrix (**a**, **b**).

Low-grade central osteosarcoma is composed of a variably cellular spindle-cell/fibroblastic proliferation that, as the name suggests, lacks the degree of cytological atypia seen in conventional osteosarcoma. Moreover, bone production within this spindle-cell proliferation appears as irregular, somewhat thick, anastomosing or branching bony trabeculae that simulate the

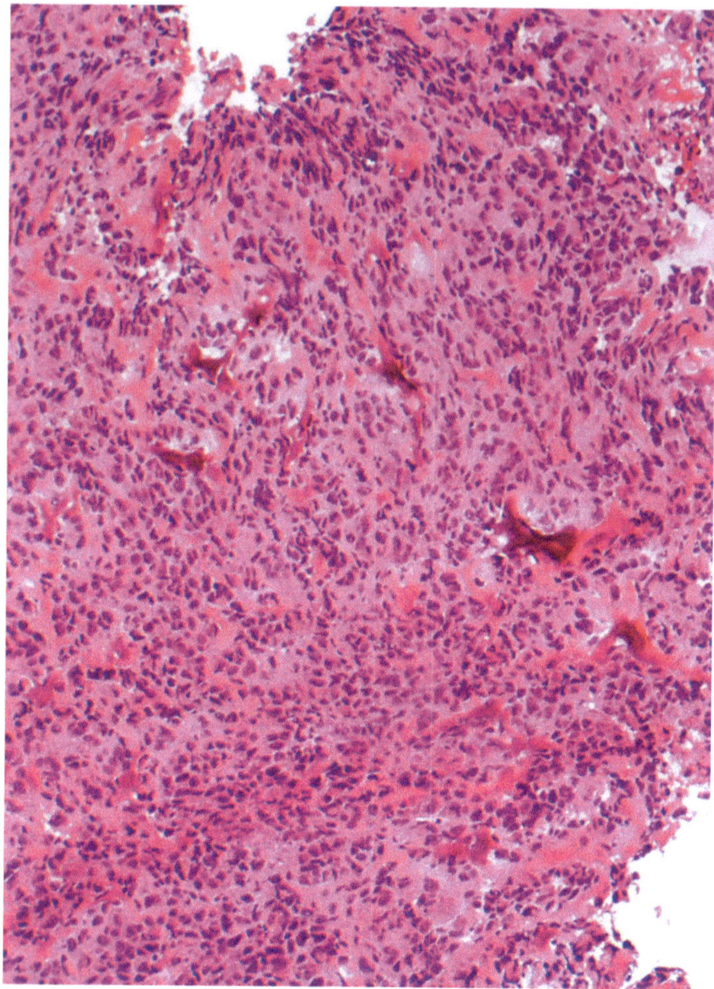

FIGURE 2.14 Hyperchromasia and nuclear atypia can be appreciated in this osteosarcoma, even at this low power.

woven bone of fibrous dysplasia, or the longitudinal seams of bone seen in parosteal osteosarcoma (see below). Although review of the radiological findings often reveals subtle signs of malignancy and helps to exclude a benign lesion such as fibrous dysplasia or desmoplastic fibroma, it is best to defer the diagnosis of this rare variant to the permanent sections.

Telangiectatic osteosarcoma is characterized by large blood-filled spaces separated by hypercellular fibrous septae that contain

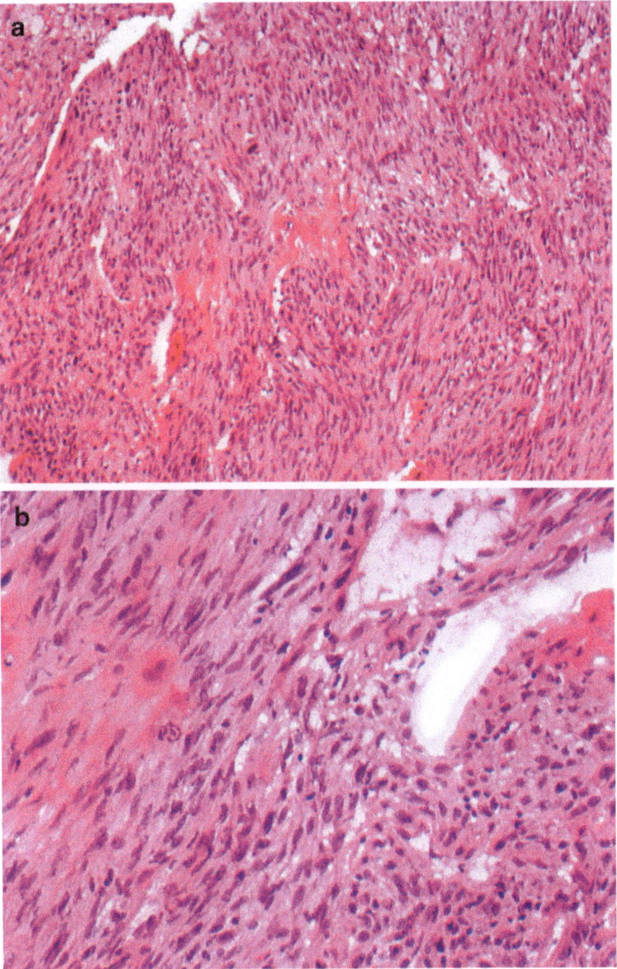

FIGURE 2.15 Some osteosarcomas can be composed almost entirely of spindle cells. Notice the osteoid in the center (**a**). Significant nuclear atypia is also present (**b**).

variable amounts of tumor osteoid and markedly pleomorphic cells. Although one might not readily see the osteoid on a single frozen section slide, the degree of pleomorphism present in the cells lining the blood lakes usually makes the diagnosis of malignancy relatively straightforward. This, along with the tumor's characteristic radiolucent and expansile appearance on radiological examination, should strongly suggest the diagnosis.

Small cell osteosarcoma histologically resembles Ewing's sarcoma, except that there is at least focal evidence (usually scant) of osteoid formation (Fig. 2.16).

In contrast to *central osteosarcomas* that arise in the medullary cavity, the much less common *surface osteosarcomas* arise on the

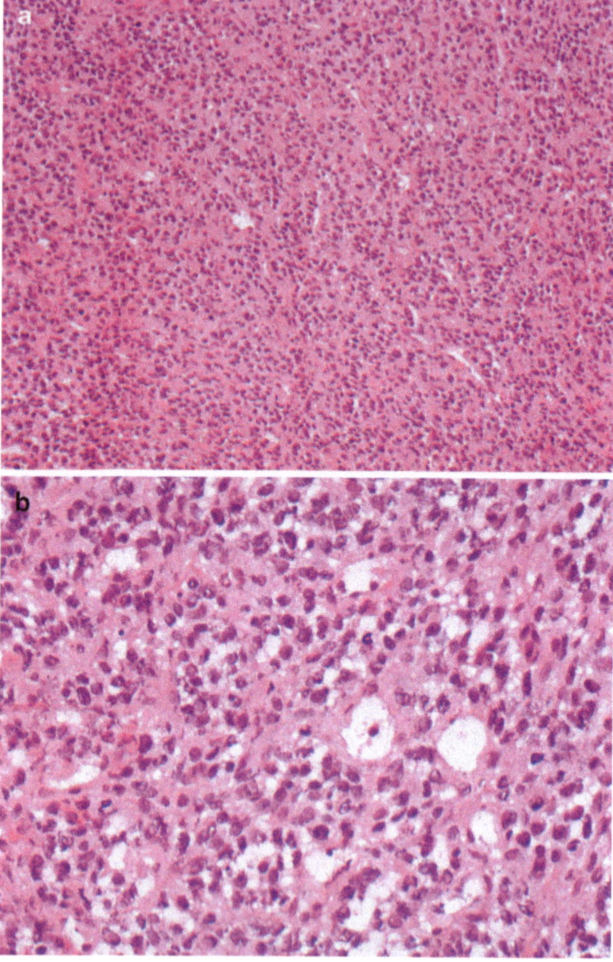

FIGURE 2.16 Small-cell osteosarcoma (**a**, **b**) may be very difficult to distinguish from other round cell tumors of bone (such as lymphoma or Ewing's sarcoma) and may not be correctly diagnosed in frozen section material unless direct osteoid production by tumor cells is identified. In this case, this was only found on permanent sections.

cortical surface. Of these, *high-grade surface osteosarcoma* is histologically identical to conventional intramedullary osteosarcoma; *parosteal osteosarcoma* (the commonest surface osteosarcoma) resembles low-grade central osteosarcoma, whereas periosteal osteosarcoma characteristically has abundant cartilaginous matrix and cytomorphologically falls between the low- and high-grade variants.

Again, it should be stressed that although awareness of the particular features of the osteosarcoma variants is useful especially to avoid a misdiagnosis, subclassification of osteosarcoma is seldom necessary on frozen section interpretation and is best deferred to permanent sections.

Chapter 3
Cartilage-Producing Lesions

INTRODUCTION

Tumors that produce a chondroid matrix are traditionally grouped together regardless of their histogenesis. There are three types of cartilage: hyaline cartilage, fibrocartilage, and elastic cartilage. In the adult, hyaline cartilage is present in the joints; fibrocartilage is mostly found in the spine; and elastic cartilage is seen in the external ear, epiglottis, and a few other places. The vast majority of cartilaginous matrix encountered in frozen sections is hyaline cartilage, which is easily recognizable based on its amorphous basophilic quality. Mature chondrocytes reside within sharp-edged lacunar spaces embedded in the matrix and have finely granular eosinophilic cytoplasm that is often vacuolated. The nuclei are typically small and round with condensed chromatin ("tight nuclei"). The nuclear detail is usually not appreciated. The presence of small clusters of chondrocytes, more than one cell per lacuna, and occasional binucleation is not uncommon. Mitotic activity is usually not discernable.

As for all bone lesions, evaluation of cartilaginous lesions necessitates adequate correlation with radiographic findings. This is extremely important during intraoperative consultation (frozen section), when the diagnosis may dictate the immediate subsequent surgical procedure, i.e., curettage with bone grafting vs. amputation. Oftentimes, conventional radiographic images are sufficient to guide the diagnosis. Computed tomography (CT) and magnetic resonance imaging (MRI) are useful in determining cortical or soft tissue involvement and possible coexistent secondary lesions [e.g., aneurysmal bone cyst (ABC)].

O. Hameed et al., *Frozen Section Library: Bone*, Frozen Section Library,
DOI 10.1007/978-1-4419-8376-3_3, © Springer Science+Business Media, LLC 2011

OSTEOCHONDROMA

Osteochondroma is the most common benign tumor of bone and is characterized by a hyaline cartilage-capped, exophytic, bony projection arising on the surface of bone. The tumor is more commonly seen in males and peaks in the second decade of life. The most common location is the metaphysis of long bones, especially around the knee. On imaging, osteochondroma demonstrates continuity of marrow and cortex with the underlying parent bone. These lesions are usually easily diagnosed by radiographic modalities with the cartilage cap pointing away from the nearest joint. However, in cases clinically concerning for malignancy (e.g., pain, rapid growth, thick and irregular cartilage cap), an open biopsy with frozen section interpretation may be performed to determine the immediate surgical strategy.

An osteochondroma may be sessile or pedunculated with a smooth and thin cartilage cap (normally <1 cm, decreasing with age). A cartilage cap of greater than 2–3 cm raises suspicion of malignant transformation. The chondrocytes in an osteochondroma are organized and undergo endochondral ossification, mimicking that of growth plate. However, these features are best appreciated in permanent sections of excisional specimens. The diagnostic challenge is mostly during frozen section interpretation, where the nature of the lesion often needs to be determined from a small biopsy specimen.

While loss of architecture, myxoid change, nuclear atypia, mitotic activity, and necrosis are all features indicative of malignant transformation, the cartilage cap in an osteochondroma may be more cellular than ordinary chondromas. Thus, the threshold of cellularity for malignancy in the setting of osteochondroma should be higher in the absence of other worrisome features (Fig. 3.1).

Although surface chondrosarcoma may be histologically indistinguishable from chondrosarcoma arising in an osteochondroma, the former is characterized by the absence of a stalk radiographically and grossly. Although a parosteal osteosarcoma may have a zone of cartilage simulating a "cap," it can be histologically separated from an osteochondroma by an atypical fibroblastic proliferation and tumor osteoid formation.

Bizarre parosteal osteochondromatous proliferation (Nora's lesion) may also be encountered in the differential diagnosis. This lesion predominantly affects small tubular bones of the hands and feet but has been well described in long bones and is not continuous with the underlying bone. Histologically, the lesion consists of seemingly random mixture of bone, cartilage, and proliferative bizarre fibroblasts and is frequently very cellular. Furthermore, the hyaline cartilage in Nora's lesion is typically disorganized, with patchy ossification, but no "columnation" of the cartilage as is seen in osteochondromas.

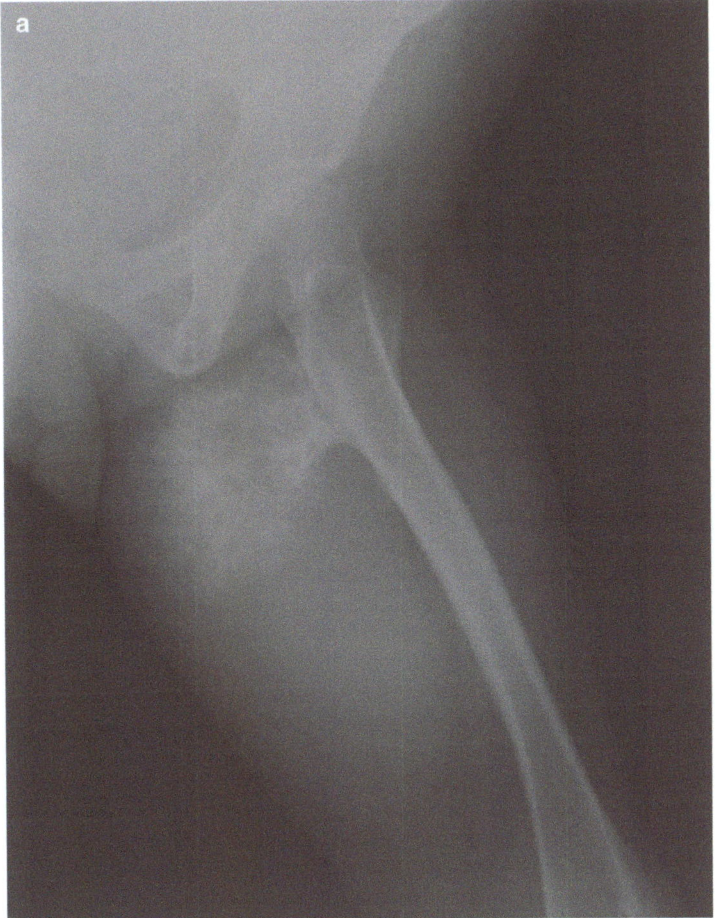

FIGURE 3.1 A 48-year-old woman, with history of multiple hereditary exostoses, presented with a large left proximal femoral mass, consistent with osteochondroma (**a**). While the frozen section shows increased cellularity in the cartilage cap, there is no significant nuclear pleomorphism, mitotic activity, or necrosis (**b**), which, in combination of the thickness of the cartilage cap (0.5 cm), warrants a diagnosis of osteochondroma.

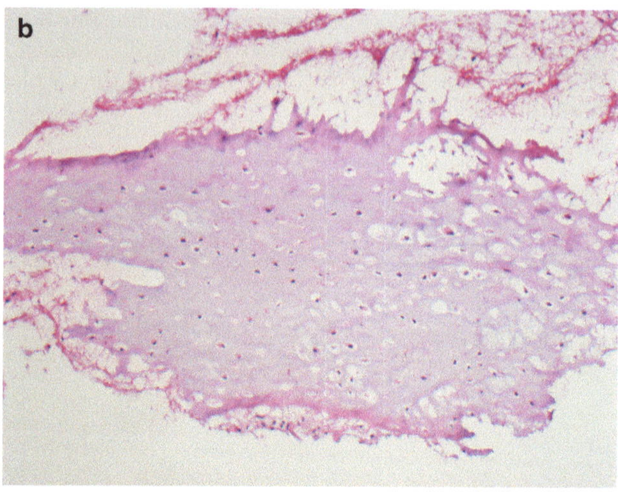

FIGURE 3.1 (continued)

CHONDROMAS

This group of benign tumors of hyaline cartilage consists of enchondroma, periosteal chondroma, and enchondromatosis. While they share many histologic features, these lesions differ with respect to location and clinical manifestation.

Enchondromas arise from the medullary cavity, with a wide age distribution, but peak in the second through fourth decades. They frequently occur in the small bones of hands and feet and may present with pain and pathologic fracture. Long bone tumors are less common and are more often asymptomatic. Radiographically, enchondromas are typically well-demarcated radiolucencies with variable amounts of mineralization. Rings and arcs or popcorn-like calcifications, when present, are the most characteristic findings. Lesions of small tubular bones may be expansile or replace the medullary cavity. In contrast, the presence of bony expansion and scalloping in long bones suggests low-grade chondrosarcoma.

Curettage specimens received for frozen section evaluation are typically pale blue or translucent hyaline cartilage fragments, which may be associated with intermixed bony spicules representing endochondral ossification. Histologically, enchondromas are typically composed of hypocellular lobules with abundant pale blue hyaline cartilage matrix, which may be associated with endochondral ossification at the periphery. The lesional cells are round to ovoid and situated within lacunae, similar to the normal chondrocytes of the growth plate. The nuclei are small and dark, and the nuclear details are usually difficult to appreciate. Binucleated forms are rare (Fig. 3.2). It should be noted that enchondromas of small bones in the hands and feet may have increased cellularity, cytologic atypia, binucleation, and myxoid change. Thus, the presence of these features should not be regarded a priori as low-grade chondrosarcoma especially if they appear nonaggressive radiographically (Fig. 3.3). On the other hand, chondrosarcomas of long

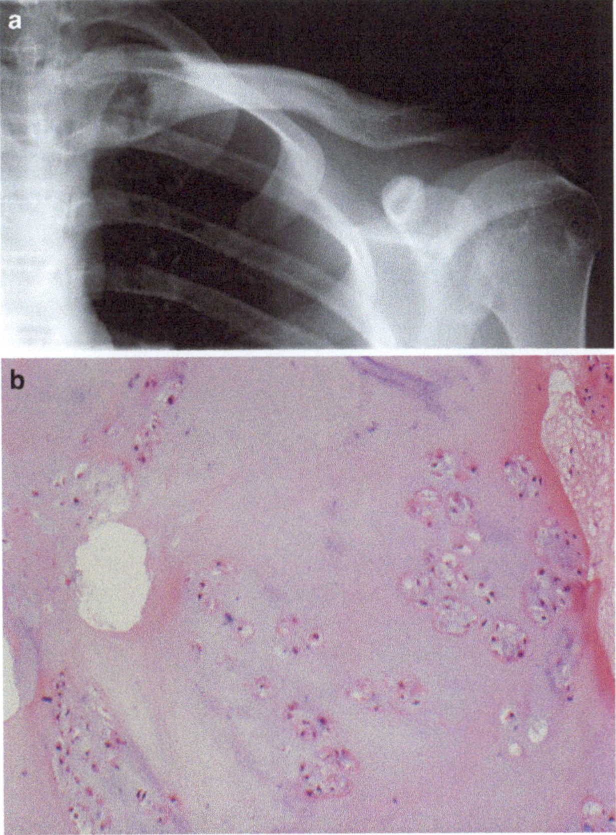

FIGURE 3.2 Enchondroma. A 14-year-old boy presented with a minimally expansile lytic lesion involving the proximal left clavicle. No obvious aggressive features are seen (**a**). The frozen section shows hypocellular lobules with abundant hyaline cartilage matrix. No atypical cytologic features are present (**b**). The findings are consistent with an enchondroma.

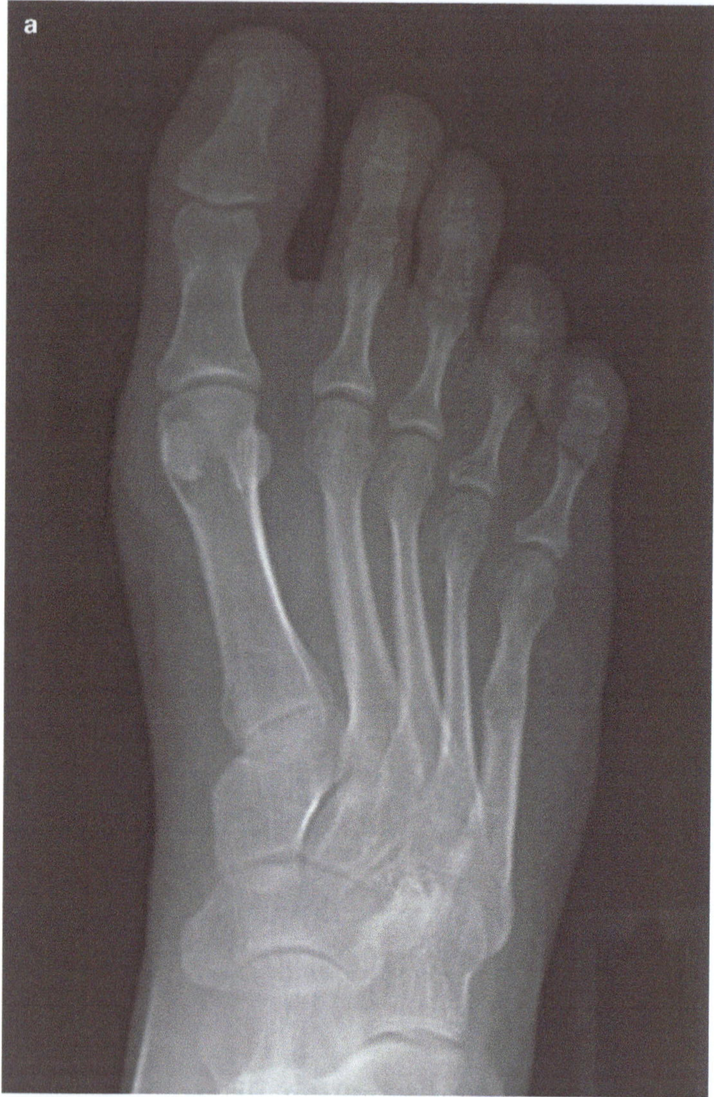

FIGURE 3.3 Enchondroma. This elongated lucent lesion in the right fifth metatarsal of a 30-year-old female has no aggressive radiographic features (**a**). The frozen section showed a hypercellular cartilage lesion with focal myxoid change (**b**), features that may otherwise represent malignancy; however, given the location and the nonaggressive appearance on imaging, the lesion is mostly consistent with enchondroma.

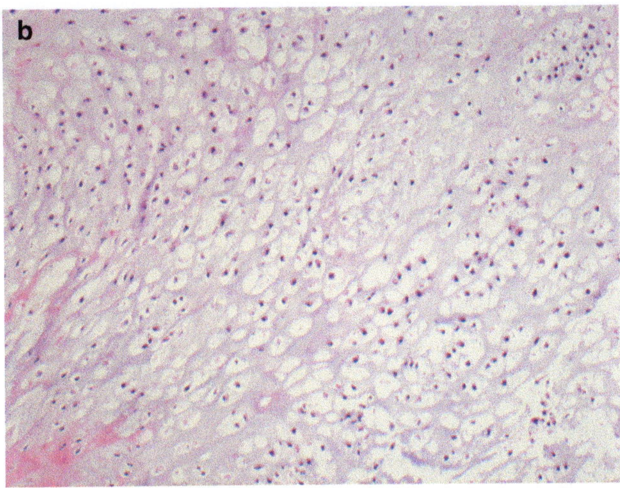

FIGURE 3.3 (continued)

bones may have hypocellular areas that mimic enchondroma. Thus, radiologic–pathologic correlation is critical in diagnosing any hyaline cartilage lesion. If radiographic information is not accessible or not provided, the diagnosis should be deferred until obtained during permanent section signout.

Periosteal chondromas (also known as juxtacortical chondroma) arise on the cortical surface and most commonly occur in the metadiaphysis of long bones (about two-thirds involve the humerus and femur). These lesions are usually small (less than 3 cm), well-circumscribed, with "saucerization" (partial cortical erosion) of the underlying bone and "buttressing" (lifted periosteum by the lesion that appears to project out from the axis of the bone) on radiographs. The gross and microscopic features of periosteal chondromas closely resemble those of enchondromas of the small bones in the hands and feet. The tumors are typically hypercellular with increased binucleated forms. Nuclear atypia may be prominent. However, the tumor does not permeate Haversian canals or the medulla. The differential diagnosis includes periosteal chondrosarcoma, periosteal osteosarcoma, and Nora's lesion. Thus, a definitive diagnosis on frozen (or permanent) sectioning cannot be rendered with certainty without radiological correlation.

Enchondromatosis is rare and mostly arises in the setting of Ollier's disease (multiple enchodromas) and Mafucci's syndrome (multiple enchondromas with associated soft tissue hemangiomas). The hand is the most common site. Both of these developmental disorders are associated with significantly increased risk of secondary chondrosarcoma. While the histological features overlap those of other cartilaginous lesions as described above, it should be noted that the enchondromas in these patients tend to be more cellular than solitary enchondromas, thus the histomorphologic appearance alone cannot always be used to assess malignant transformation.

CHONDROBLASTOMA

Chondroblastoma is a rare, benign cartilage-producing tumor that mostly affects skeletally immature patients. Most patients are between 10 and 25 years of age, with a slight male predominance. It usually arises in the epiphysis (or apophysis) of long bones, most commonly around the knee, and in the proximal humerus. The skull may also be involved but usually at an older age.

Radiographically, chondroblastoma is typically a small and sharply demarcated lytic lesion with a sclerotic rim (Fig. 3.4). Spotty matrix calcifications may also be present. The lesion may extend into the metaphysis. The classic microscopic findings of chondroblastoma at lower magnification include randomly distributed osteoclast-type multinucleated giant cells and variably sized, amorphous or eosinophilic fibrochondroid islands that may be focally calcified. Calcification may take the form of a fine network of pericellular highlighting (so-called "chicken wire" calcification). At higher magnification, the cellular component consists of oval, polygonal mononuclear cells (chondroblasts) with well-defined cell borders and eosinophilic cytoplasm. The nuclei have longitudinal grooves, resulting in a "coffee bean" appearance (Fig. 3.4) similar to that of the principle cells in Langerhans cell histiocytosis (LCH). Mitotic activity may be present but is usually low (<3/10 high power fields). True hyaline cartilage is almost

FIGURE 3.4 Chondroblastoma. A 14-year-old young man presented with hip pain. Conventional radiographs demonstrated a lucent lesion in the developing apophysis of the left greater trochanter with sclerotic margins (**a**). There is no periosteal reaction. The radiographic differential diagnosis includes chondroblastoma and osteoblastoma. On frozen sections, the tissue contains fibrochondroid islands and "chicken wire"-type pericellular calcifications (**b**), as well as sheets of polygonal mononuclear cells with well-defined cell borders and eosinophilic cytoplasm (**c**). The findings are characteristic of a chondroblastoma.

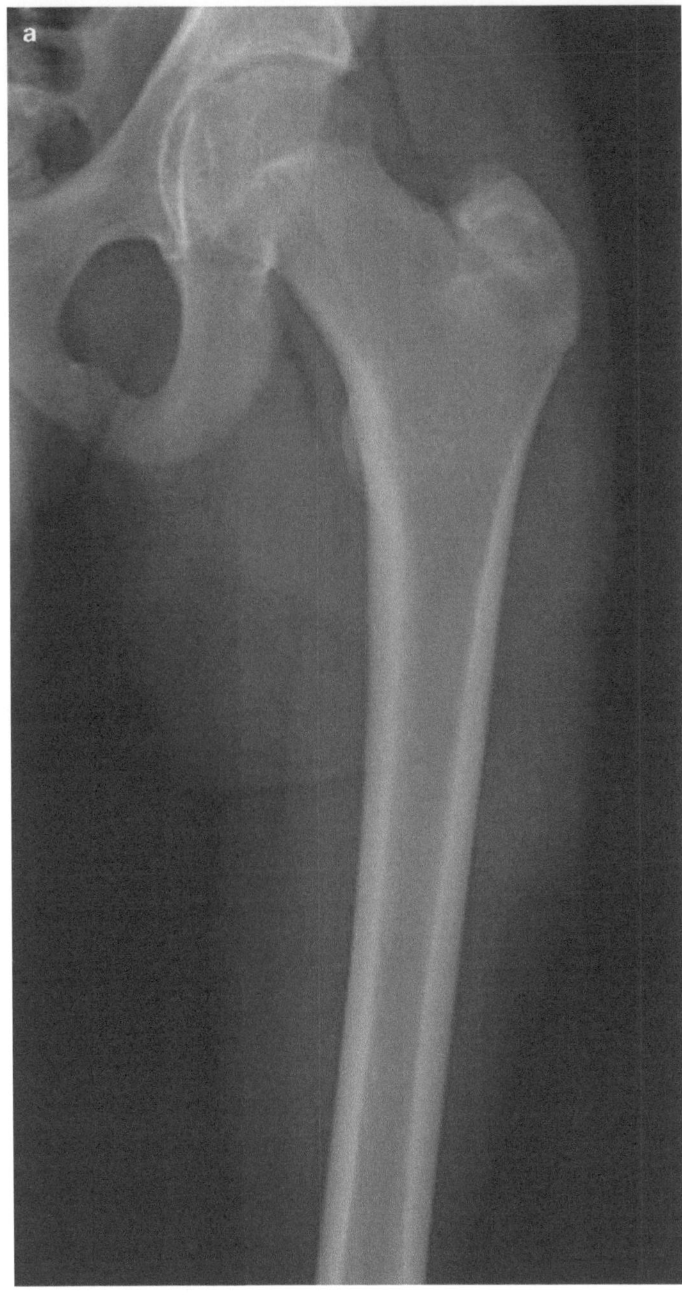

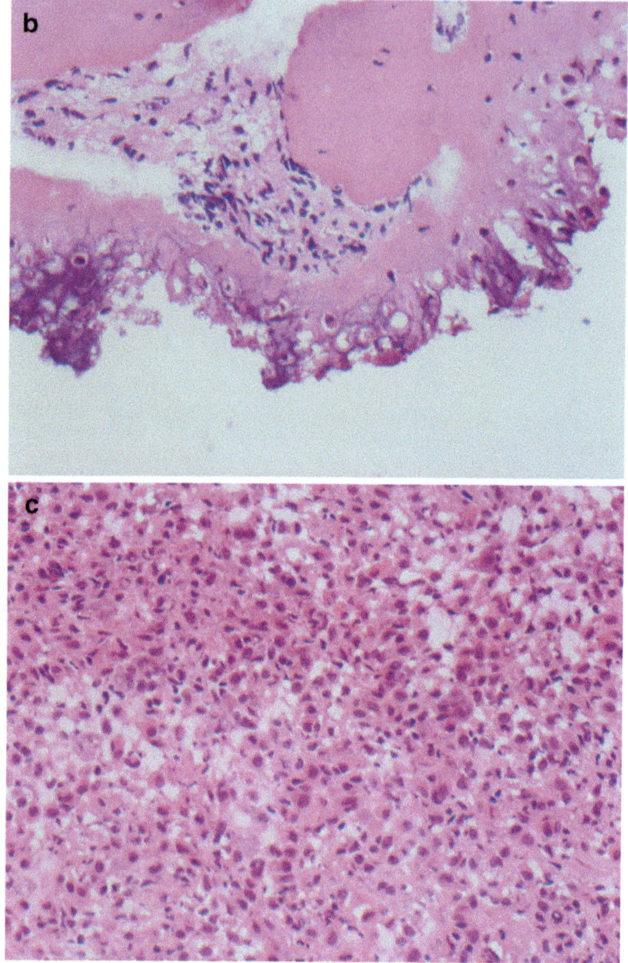

FIGURE 3.4 (continued)

never found. It is important to note that such lesions may show varying degrees of the aforementioned features, but only a small proportion of cases demonstrates all of the histologic characteristics, especially during frozen section evaluation, as the material is often limited and/or detailed microscopic examination is hindered by prominent calcification.

The histologic differential diagnosis of chondroblastoma includes giant cell tumor (GCT) of bone, chondromyxoid fibroma

(CMF), LCH, and ABC. GCT (Chap. 5) is seldom seen in skeletally immature individuals. Histologically, the GCT typically shows numerous, evenly distributed osteoclast-like giant cells in a background of mononuclear cells with similar appearing nuclei. CMF (next entity) typically occurs in the metaphysis and consists of zonated lobules of spindled and stellate cells in a background of myxoid stroma. LCH (Chap. 6) has a predilection for flat bone involvement and typically shows a variety of inflammatory cells (especially eosinophils). The Langerhans cells may mimic chondroblasts, but the lesion typically lacks matrix formation and calcifications. ABC (Chap. 5) may occur anywhere within the bone, although primary ABC usually spares the epiphysis. CT or MRI, if performed preoperatively, typically shows fluid–fluid levels. Although the presence of osteoclast-like giant cells and basophilic calcifications overlaps with chondroblastoma, the presence of blood-filled spaces and fibroblastic proliferation along with the absence of sheets of chondroblasts should help point to the diagnosis of ABC. It should be noted, however, that secondary ABC commonly coexists with chondroblastoma. Thus, care should be taken when features of ABC are seen in a specimen from an epiphyseal lesion or when radiographic information is not provided. In such cases, communication with the surgeon is imperative prior to providing the diagnosis.

CHONDROMYXOID FIBROMA

CMF is one of the least common tumors of bone. It has a wide age range but peaks in the second and third decades. In its typical presentation, CMF occurs in the intramedullary portion of the metaphysis of long bones, most commonly in the proximal tibia. Imaging studies typically show sharp, sclerotic margins with scalloping. Matrix calcification is rare, except when present in the juxtacortical location.

Histologically, the lesion has a vaguely lobular pattern caused by hypocelluar centers and increased cellularity at the periphery. The lobules are composed of varying proportions of fibrous, myxomatous, and chondroid tissue containing spindled and stellate cells which are more zonally numerous at the periphery of the lobules. Osteoclast-like giant cells are also often present at the periphery. Well-formed hyaline cartilage is only rarely present. It should be noted that the zonated configuration of CMF may not be well preserved in the limited frozen material sent for examination, especially when the curetting specimen is largely fragmented. The myxoid matrix may appear edematous and mimic freezing artifact (Fig. 3.5).

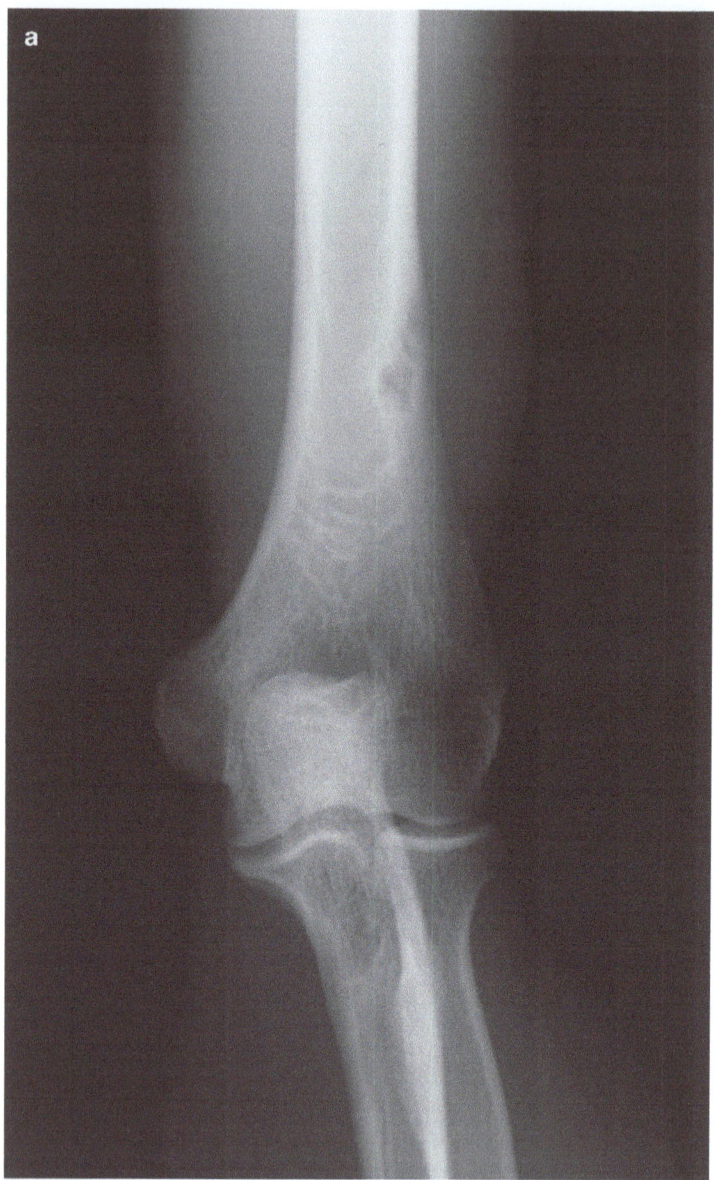

FIGURE 3.5 Chondromyxoid fibroma. There is an eccentric osteolytic lesion in the distal humerus of this 53-year-old man which involves the lateral cortex (**a**). Frozen sections of the curettage specimen revealed spindled and stellate cells embedded in somewhat myxoid matrix that mimics edema or freezing artifact (**b**). The cells are arranged in a lobulated pattern with increased cellularity at the periphery. Although cortical involvement is not a common finding, the histologic features are typical for chondromyxoid fibroma.

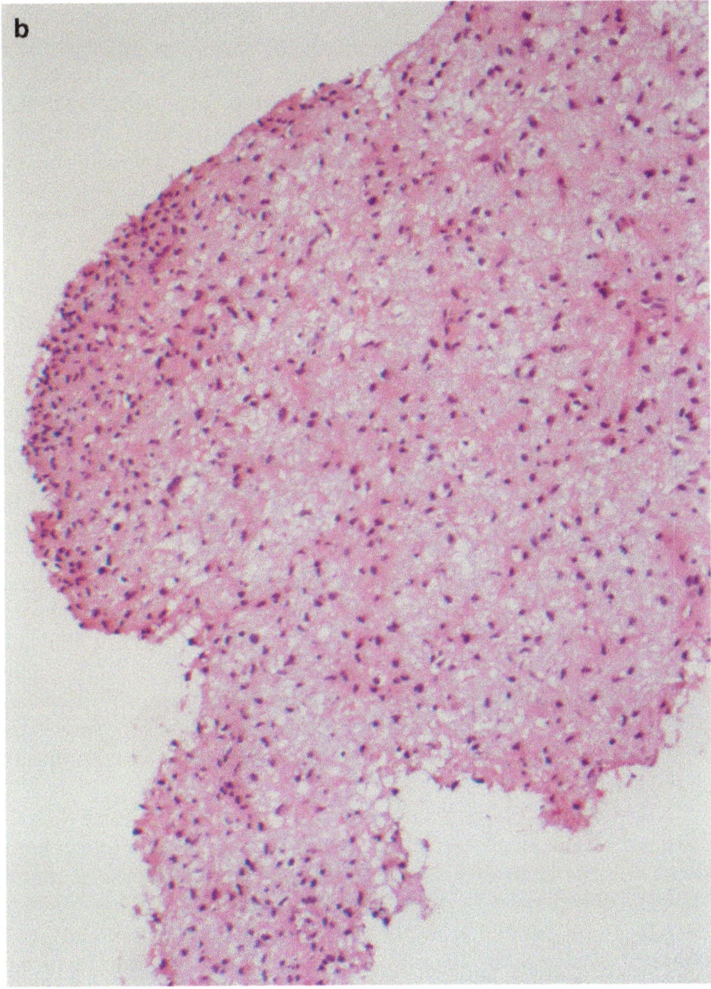

FIGURE 3.5 (continued)

The cytomorphology of CMF may mimic chondroblast-oma. However, the latter occurs almost exclusively in the epi-physis and histologically does not have lobular configuration. Chondroma is also a differential diagnostic consideration but usually can be excluded by the presence of predominant hyaline cartilage. Chondroblastic osteosarcoma may have overlapping histolomorphology with CMF especially as related to the matrix. Chondroblastic osteosarcoma, however, typically demonstrates an aggressive radiographic appearance and the presence of, at least focally, hyaline cartilage and tumor-producing osteoid. Chondro-sarcoma usually occurs in the older patients and can be excluded by the presence of permeation of bone radiographically and microscopically.

CHONDROSARCOMA

Chondrosarcoma is the second most common malignant neoplasm of bone. The tumor usually occurs in adults and peaks between the fifth and sixth decades. Chondrosarcoma may affect any bone; the most frequent sites of involvement include the bones of the pelvis, proximal femur, and rib. Rarely, the tumor arises de novo in extraskeletal sites. On imaging, chondrosarcoma typically presents as a rapidly growing, large radiolucency with punctate or ring-like calcifications and cortical erosion (scalloping). Cortical disruption and soft tissue extension may be seen in advanced lesions (Figs. 3.6 and 3.7).

The fresh tissue of chondrosarcoma received for frozen sectioning is typically pale blue with a mucoid or myxoid matrix. A lobular growth pattern may be appreciated in a larger specimen but is replaced by sheet-like growth in high-grade lesions. Chalky white calcium deposits are commonly present. Microscopically, the tumor grows in nodules separated by fibrous bands and produces abundant blue-gray cartilaginous matrix on H&E staining.

Conventional chondrosarcoma varies in cellularity from field to field but is typically hypercellular when compared with an enchondroma of the same site. The chondrocytes are variable in size and shape accompanied by hyperchromasia and discernible nuclear details ("open-nuclei"); binucleation is also frequent. Myxoid changes and matrix liquefaction are other common features, whereas necrosis and atypical mitoses are rare and indicative of a high-grade lesion. Another important feature to distinguish chondrosarcoma from enchondroma is permeation through the cortex or invasion and overrunning of the bone trabeculae in the medulla. It should be noted that endochondral ossification is commonly seen at the periphery of tumor lobules and should not dissuade one from the diagnosis of chondrosarcoma if all the other features are present. On the other hand, the identification of tumor osteoid or bone formation directly by tumor cells should point to the diagnosis of (chondroblastic) osteosarcoma, rather than chondrosarcoma.

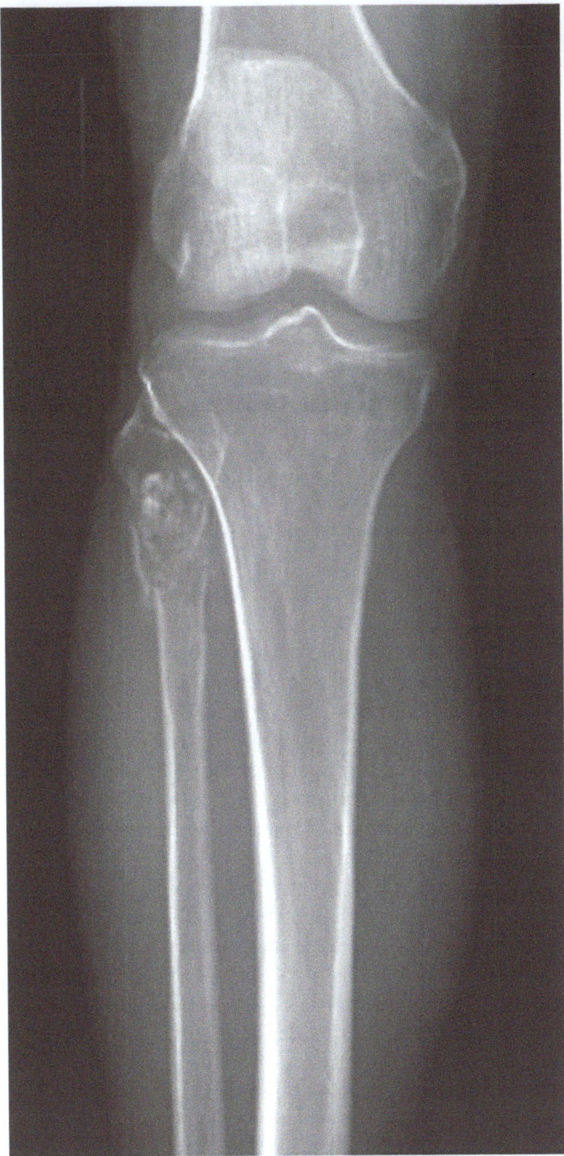

FIGURE 3.6 Chondrosarcoma. The conventional radiograph shows a centrally placed lesion in the proximal fibula of a 59-year-old man. The lesion contains chondroid matrix and demonstrates endosteal scalloping with associated pathologic fracture. The most likely consideration is a low-grade chondrosarcoma.

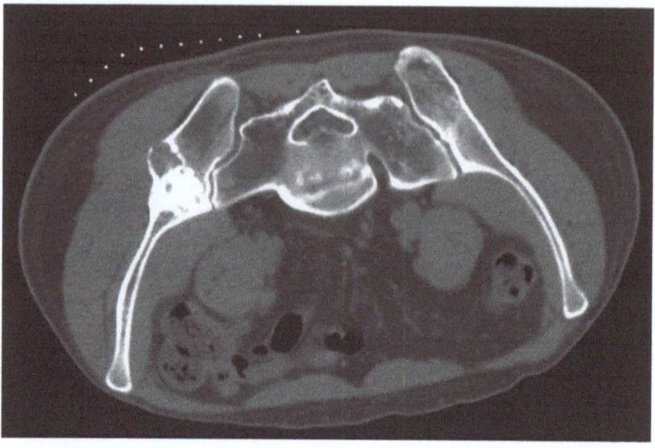

FIGURE 3.7   A CT scan showing a 4.5 cm mixed densely sclerotic and lytic right iliac wing lesion with cortical breakthrough, concerning for chondrosarcoma versus osteosarcoma or less likely a metastatic lesion. The histologic sections demonstrated a grade II chondrosarcoma.

Given that increased cellularity, binucleation, hyperchromasia, and myxoid change all may be seen in enchondromas of the small bones of hands, only the presence of unequivocal radiologic or histologic evidence of tumor permeation through the cortex can the diagnosis of chondrosarcoma in these locations be made. Conversely, one should also bear in mind that curettage specimens do not always have preserved geographic relationships maintained with the adjacent bony structures, and lack of permeation in the histologic sections examined (frozen or permanent) does not automatically exclude malignancy.

Grading is most useful to predict clinical outcome in chondrosarcoma, except for those arising in the bones of the fingers and toes. Nevertheless, accurate assessment is also critical during frozen section diagnosis, as it often determines the subsequent management. Chondrosarcoma is graded on a scale of I–III, primarily based on cellularity, nuclear size and details, as popularized by Evans. However, other competing systems exist yielding no universally accepted strict scoring system.

- *Grade I*: similar to enchondroma except mildly increased cellularity, occasional binucleation and hyperchromasia, and permeative growth pattern (Fig. 3.8).
- *Grade II*: increased cellularity, myxoid changes, cytologic atypia including visible nuclear detail, hyperchromasia, and frequent binucleation (Fig. 3.9).

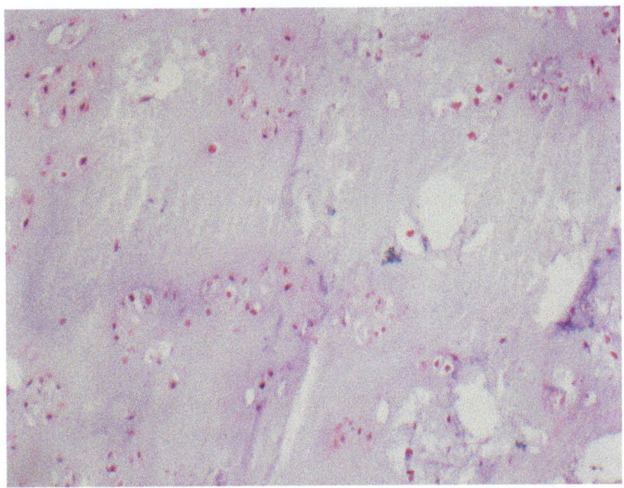

FIGURE 3.8 An example of grade I chondrosarcoma of a long bone as seen on frozen section. Note the mildly increased cellularity and binucleated forms but minimal nuclear atypia that overlap substantially with enchondroma. However, the myxoid changes and chondroid matrix liquefaction are common features of chondrosarcoma.

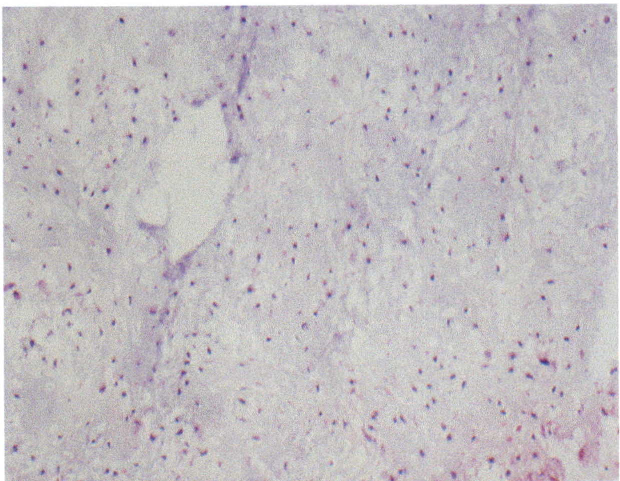

FIGURE 3.9 Grade II chondrosarcoma. In addition to myxoid changes, note the markedly increased cellularity, cellular pleomorphism, and hyperchromasia that are appreciated even at intermediate magnification.

- *Grade III*: high cellularity, significant nuclear pleomorphism; mitoses and/or necrosis may be present (Fig. 3.10).

It should be emphasized that high-grade chondrosarcomas (grade II and III) often have low-grade areas. This is particularly important in frozen section evaluation when only limited amounts of tissue are made available for histologic evaluation. Thus, when facing a radiographically aggressive lesion but no histologic evidence of malignancy, it is appropriate to defer the frozen section diagnosis. An example of how we report such a case is as follows: "cellular cartilaginous lesion, further diagnosis deferred to permanent section." On the other hand, sometimes cartilaginous lesions may represent some worrisome radiographic features (e.g., large size) but are not associated with apparent aggressive characteristics (e.g., scalloping, cortical breakthrough), and the histologic features may be similarly borderline. Again, deferral is appropriate in such a case (Figs. 3.11 and 3.12).

The histologic caveats for diagnosing periosteal chondrosarcoma (arising on surface of bone) and secondary chondrosarcoma (arising in a benign precursor, either osteochondroma or enchondroma, or in Ollier disease or Maffucci syndrome) are similar to those of conventional chondrosarcoma.

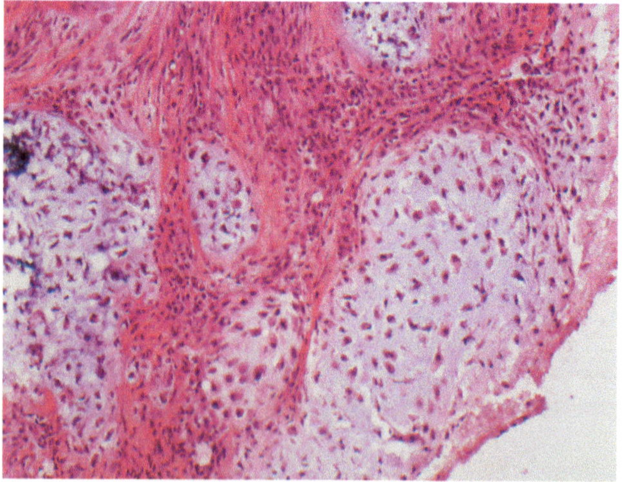

FIGURE 3.10 Grade III chondrosarcoma. Note the infiltrative growth pattern, diffuse hypercellularity, and significant pleomorphism including hyperchromasia, irregular nuclear membrane, and visible nuclear details.

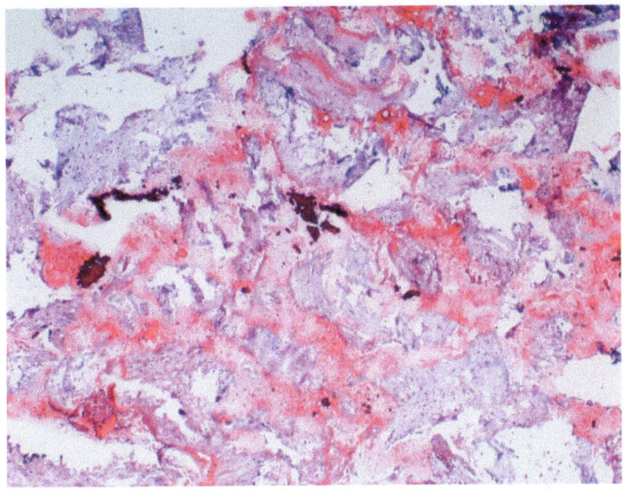

FIGURE 3.11 Borderline cartilage tumor. The curetting specimen was from a proximal humeral lesion in a 59-year-old woman. The radiologist noted a 7 cm intramedullary cartilagenous lesion with no apparent aggressive features. Frozen sections showed moderately cellular hyaline cartilage intermixed with bone dust. There was no significant nuclear pleomorphism, hyperchromasia, or mitotic activity. The radiologic findings and histomorphologic features (frozen and permanent) did not fulfill those either for an enchondroma or a low-grade chondrosarcoma. A diagnosis of "cartilaginous tumor of indeterminate biological potential" was eventually rendered, and close clinical follow-up was recommended.

CHONDROSARCOMA VARIANTS

Dedifferentiated chondrosarcoma is characterized by a bimorphic lesion composed of a well-differentiated cartilage tumor (enchondroma or low-grade chondrosarcoma) juxtaposed to a high-grade, noncartilaginous sarcoma. The radiographic findings are also commonly biphasic, with a more "aggressive" component superimposed on what is otherwise typical of chondrosarcoma. Grossly, both components are usually easily identified. The cartilaginous portion (often centrally located) is blue-gray and lobulated, and the high-grade component commonly has a soft fleshy consistency with hemorrhage and necrosis. However, the abrupt transition may not be appreciated in a frozen specimen obtained from curettings.

On histologic sections, there is similarly a distinct zone of abutment where the two components are interface. The

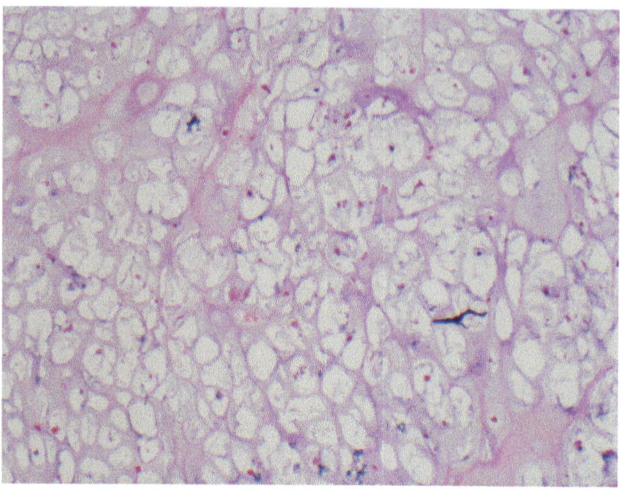

FIGURE 3.12 Similarly, this frozen section was from a mass arising from a sessile osteochondroma with a cartilage cap whose maximum thickness was 2.5 cm. The section shows prominently cellular cartilage with mild-to-moderate pleomorphism and hyperchromasia that may otherwise indicate a grade II chondrosarcoma in a long bone. However, given that the cartilage cap within an osteochondroma often shows higher cellularity and a degree of cytologic atypia greater than that of a cartilage tumor elsewhere, the diagnosis was deferred to permanent sectioning and a final diagnosis of "cartilaginous tumor of indeterminate biological potential" was rendered.

dedifferentiated area may have features of malignant fibrous histiocytoma (most frequent), osteosarcoma, fibrosarcoma, and/or rhabdomyosarcoma (Fig. 3.13). It should be noted that although by definition the dedifferentiated component is a high-grade sarcoma, we have experienced two cases where the noncartilage portion represented a predominantly giant cell-rich lesion reminiscent of a cytologically atypical GCT of bone. Thus, in our opinion, the presence of any "high-grade" mesenchymal component in association with a separate "low-grade" cartilage tumor would raise the possibility that this lesion was a dedifferentiated chondrosarcoma. Dedifferentiated chondrosarcoma is highly aggressive and has a poor prognosis.

Mesenchymal chondrosarcoma is a rare variant of chondrosarcoma that affects younger patients with a peak incidence in the second and the third decades of life. This highly malignant tumor is characterized by a bimorphic appearance in which islands of

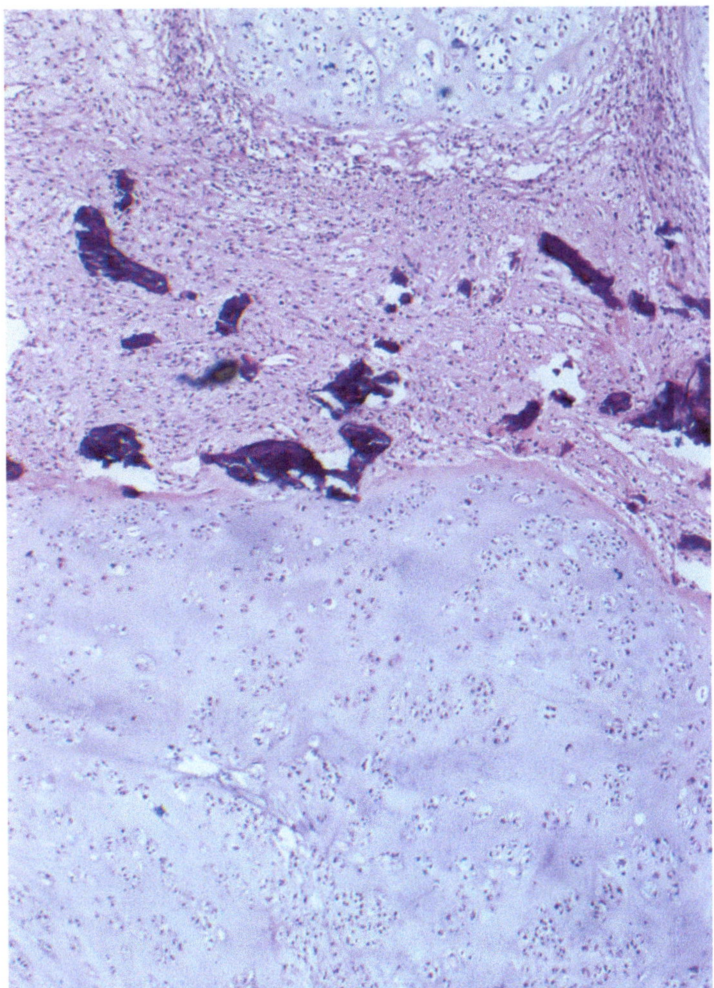

FIGURE 3.13 Dedifferentiated chondrosarcoma. The frozen section was made from tissue derived from a chest wall mass of a patient with hereditary multiple exostoses. Note the abrupt transition of a high-grade osteosarcoma (center) from the adjacent conventional relatively low-grade chondrosarcoma, most likely representing its dedifferentiated component.

mostly bland-appearing hyaline cartilage are embedded within solid, hypercellular areas of primitive small, round, blue cells (simulating Ewing sarcoma) commonly arranged in a hemangiopericytoma-like pattern (Fig. 3.14).

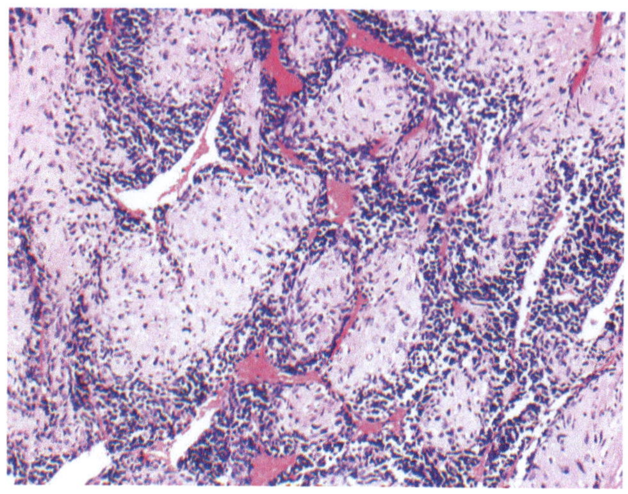

FIGURE 3.14 A section of mesenchymal chondrosarcoma with characteristic bimorphic appearance consisting of islands of hyaline cartilage and solid, hypercellular areas of primitive small, round, blue cells. Note that the cartilage in mesenchymal condrosarcoma appears benign because it represents all stages of chondrogenesis that are seen in the growth plate.

Clear cell chondrosarcoma is a rare, low-grade variant of chondrosarcoma with a predilection for the epiphyseal region of long bones. It also affects a younger age group than conventional chondrosarcoma and peaks in the third decade. Approximately two-thirds of lesions involve either the femoral or the humeral heads. The tumor consists primarily of plump cells with large, centrally located nuclei with a clear-to-pale eosinophilic cytoplasm and well-defined cell borders. Zones of low-grade chondrosarcoma, formation of woven bone and osteoclast-like multinucleated giant cells are variably present. Areas of aneurysmal bone cyst are often also identified.

Chapter 4
Fibrous and Fibrohistiocytic Lesions

INTRODUCTION

Most tumors of fibrous and fibrohistiocytic origin generally produce collagen but do not form a mineralizing matrix, whereas high-grade tumors may have little to no matrix. Fibro-osseous lesions [fibrous dysplasia (FD) and osteofibrous dysplasia (OFD)] are composed of large volumes of fibrous connective tissue, principally collagens type I and III, as well as osseous areas. Fibrous and fibrohistiocytic lesions span the entire spectrum of clinical behaviors: benign, locally aggressive, and malignant. While with radiologic input, it is usually not difficult to distinguish the benign and malignant ends of the spectrum, some of these lesions have significant overlapping histologic features and necessitate incorporating clinical and demographic information to arrive at the correct diagnosis.

NONOSSIFYING FIBROMA (METAPHYSEAL FIBROUS DEFECT)

Nonossifying fibromas (NOFs) are exclusively seen in young patients with an age range of 5–20 years. It is extremely unusual to see an NOF in individuals with fused growth plates. The most common site is the metaphysis around the knee (distal femur and proximal tibia). It is still debatable whether NOF represents a true neoplasm. Hence, some authorities prefer to use the term *metaphyseal fibrous defect* (MFD).

NOFs are mostly asymptomatic and typically incidental findings. Patients may present with a pathologic fracture if lesions are larger. Radiography they typically show an eccentric, sharply circumscribed, purely lucent, expansile process in the metaphysis of

47

O. Hameed et al., *Frozen Section Library: Bone*, Frozen Section Library,
DOI 10.1007/978-1-4419-8376-3_4, © Springer Science+Business Media, LLC 2011

a long bone. The lesion may appear multilocular and has a scalloped border and a narrow rim of marginal sclerosis (Fig. 4.1a). The association of multiple NOFs with café-au-lait skin patches has been named *Jaffe–Campanacci syndrome.*

Curetted fragments of lesional tissue are fibrous and fleshy and may vary from tan yellow to brown in color, depending on the proportions of fibrous tissue, lipid-laden histiocytes and hemosiderin deposition/hemorrhage in association with the stroma. Histologically, NOFs typically show a highly cellular spindle cell proliferation arranged in a characteristic storiform pattern in a background of collagenized stroma (Fig. 4.1b). The pattern may vary from area to area. Multinucleated giant cells are scattered throughout the lesion and thus may share many microscopic features with giant cell tumors of bone (Fig. 4.1c). However, the giant cells in NOFs are generally smaller and contain fewer nuclei than the giant cells in giant cell tumors. Lipid-laden foamy histiocytes are almost always present and so is hemosiderin deposition. On higher magnification, the spindled cells are fibroblastic in nature, without significant pleomorphism. Mitotic figures may be present but no atypical forms are seen. Reactive new bone formation is not an uncommon finding, especially at the periphery of the lesion or if pathologic fracture is present. Rarely, a superimposed secondary aneurysmal bone cyst (ABC) may occur and is clinically manifested as a rapidly enlarged mass (Fig. 4.2). This may lead to a diagnostic challenge and careful radiologic–pathologic correlation is required.

FIGURE 4.1   Nonossifying fibroma. This lesion was from a 13-year-old boy, which demonstrated a multilocular, expansile, lytic lesion in the distal fibula, with a scalloped border and a sclerotic margin. The radiologic features are those of a typical nonossifying fibroma (**a**). Microscopically, the lesion consists of cellular spindle cell proliferation in a storiform fashion (**b**) with Scattered multinucleated giant cells and scattered or clustered foamy histiocytes are typical (**c**). These cells, mimicking those seen in giant cell tumor of bone, may be misinterpreted as freezing artifacts.

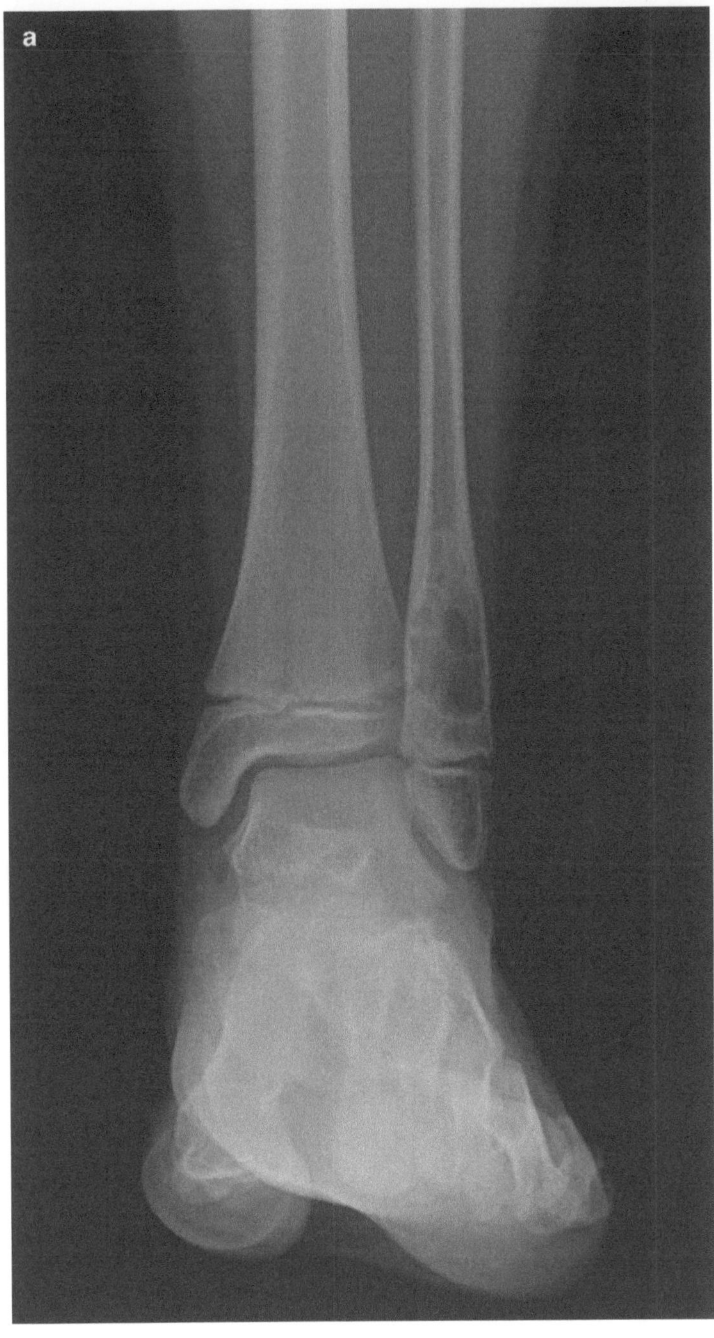
a

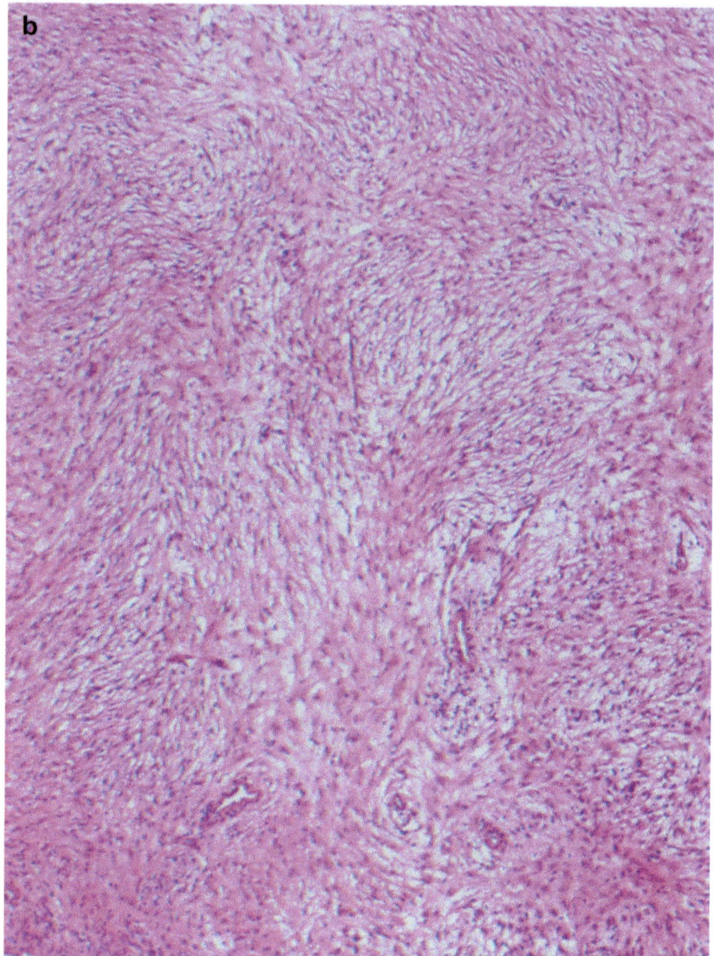

FIGURE 4.1 (continued)

BENIGN FIBROUS HISTIOCYTOMA

Benign fibrous histiocytoma (BFH) of bone is histologically indistinguishable from NOF, being separated from the latter only on clinical and radiological grounds. BFH may affect any bone, occur at any age, and present with local pain even in the absence of pathologic fracture.

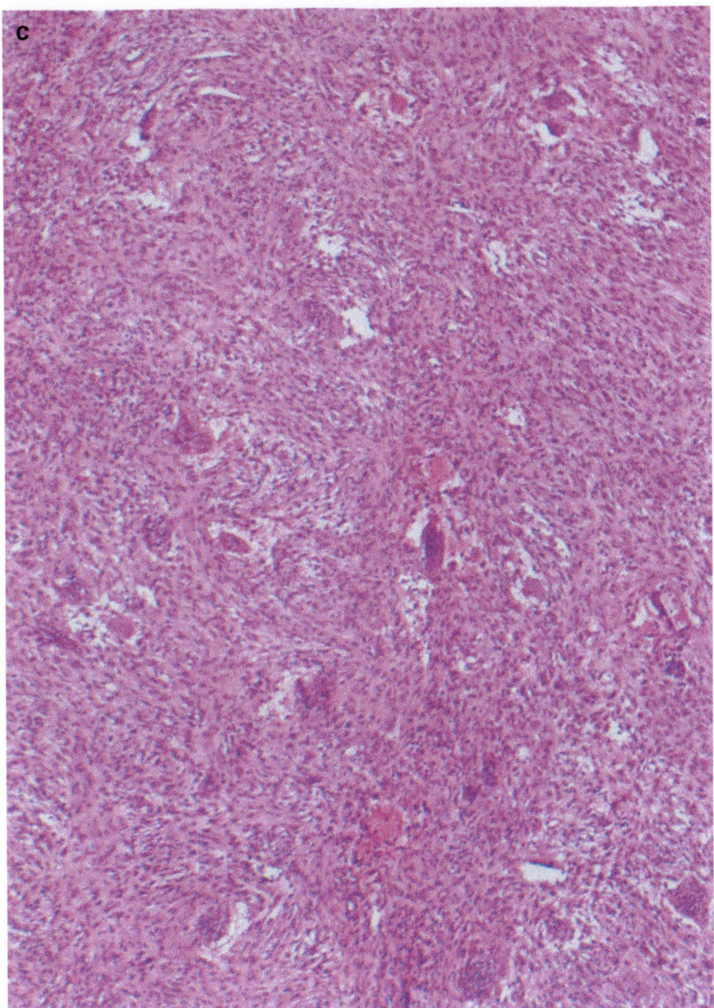

FIGURE 4.1 (continued)

Radiographically, BFH typically has a sharp margin, often with a sclerotic rim such as NOF, but may also lack a well-defined margin, destroy the cortex, and extend into soft tissue, thus mimicking a malignant process (Fig. 4.3a). When a lesion with histologic features of NOF (Fig. 4.3b, c) is seen in a skeletally mature

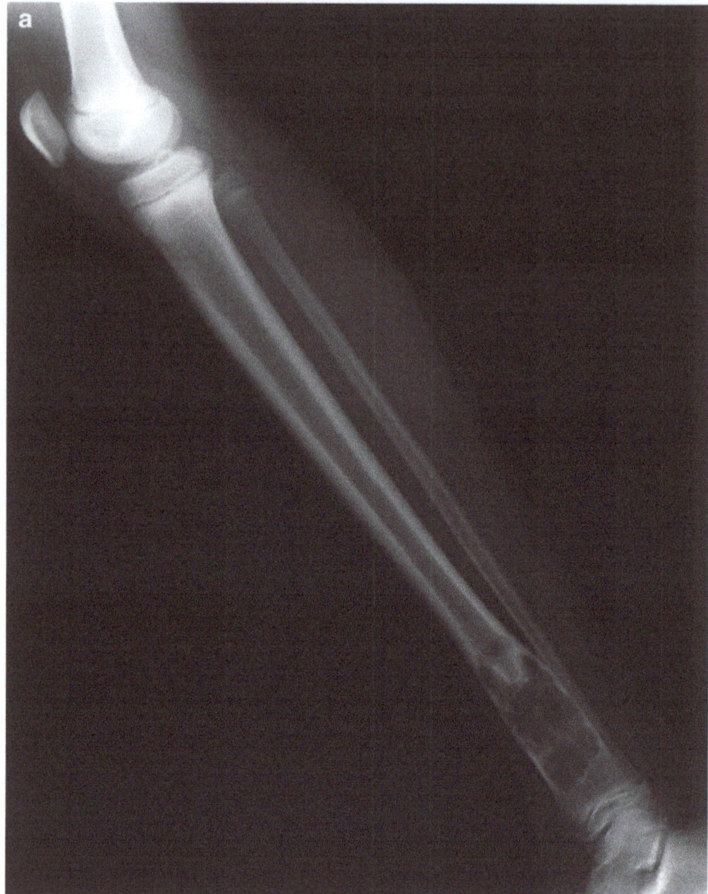

FIGURE 4.2 Nonossifying fibroma. This is a large (8.3 cm), multilocu-lated, cystic lesion in the distal tibial metaphysis of another 13-year-old boy. There are multiple internal bony septations (**a**). Histologic sections show a cellular spindle cell lesion with a storiform growth pattern and scattered giant cells, features of those of a typical nonossifying fibroma (**b**). However, a cyst wall with no apparent lining (*right upper corner*) is present, with new bone formation in a lace-like pattern in parallel to the cyst wall. The histologic features, along with the radiologic findings, are mostly consistent with a nonossifying fibroma with secondary aneurysmal bone cyst formation.

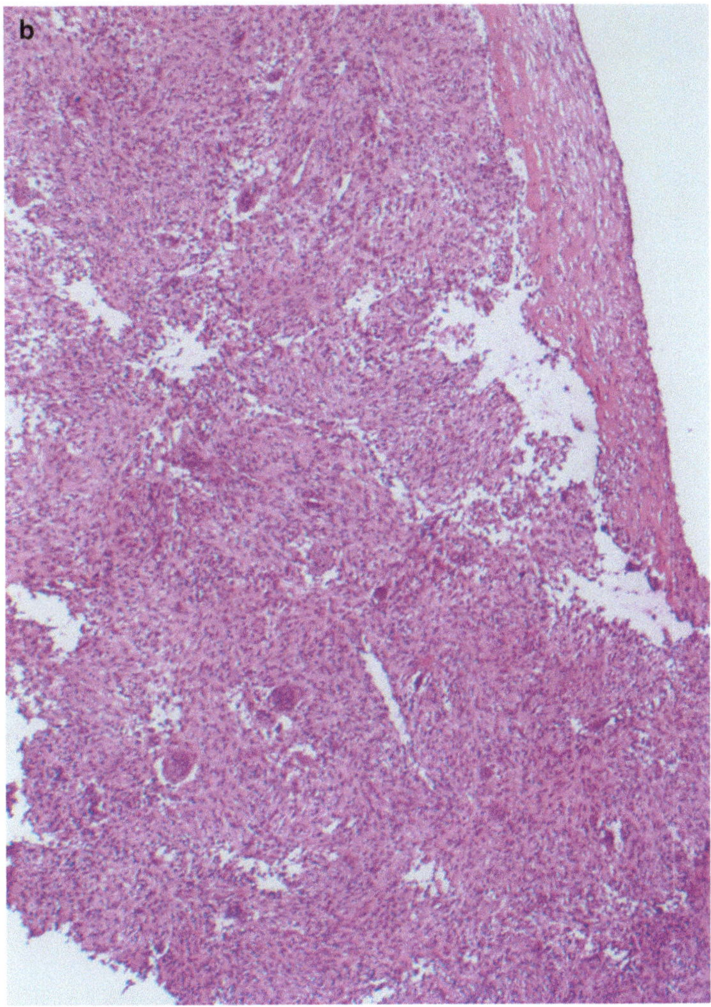

FIGURE 4.2 (continued)

patient, in a location other than metaphysis of a long bone or with associated local pain, the diagnosis of BFH is appropriate.

The differential diagnosis of NOF/BFH includes desmoplastic fibroma of bone (intra-osseous counterpart of soft tissue fibromatosis). This lesion tends to occur in younger patients, may involve any bone but is most frequent in the mandible. Radiographically, it is usually a well-defined, radiolucent lesion. If large, the lesion

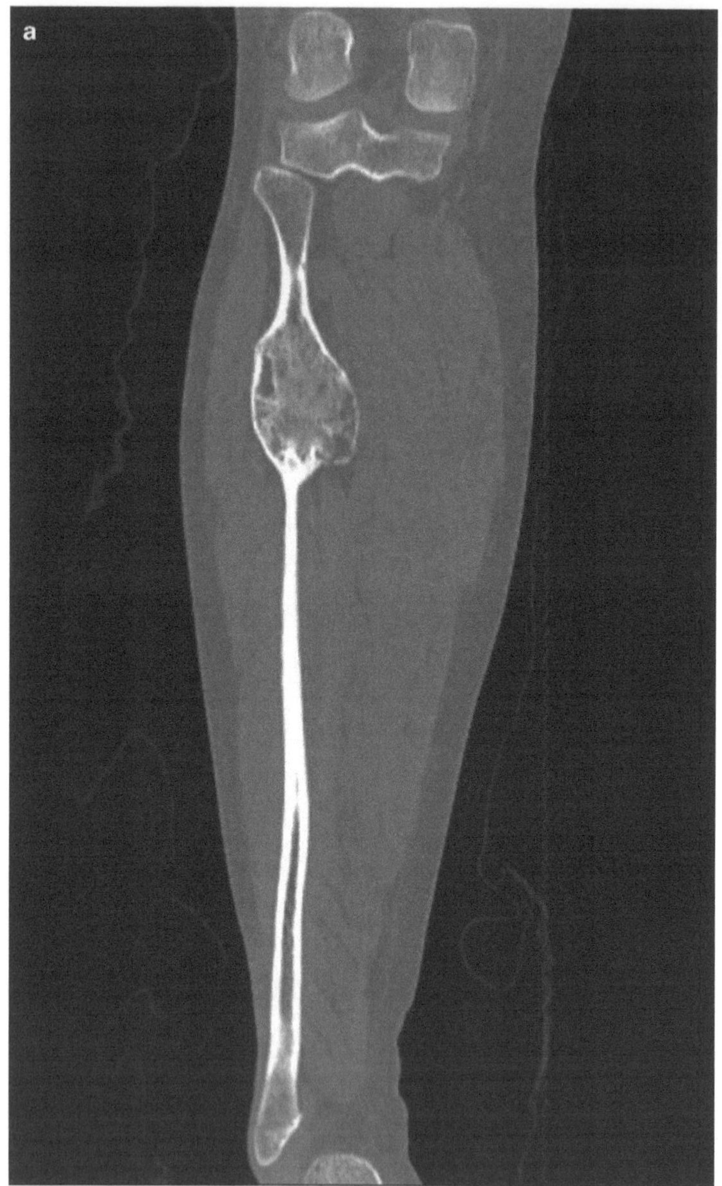

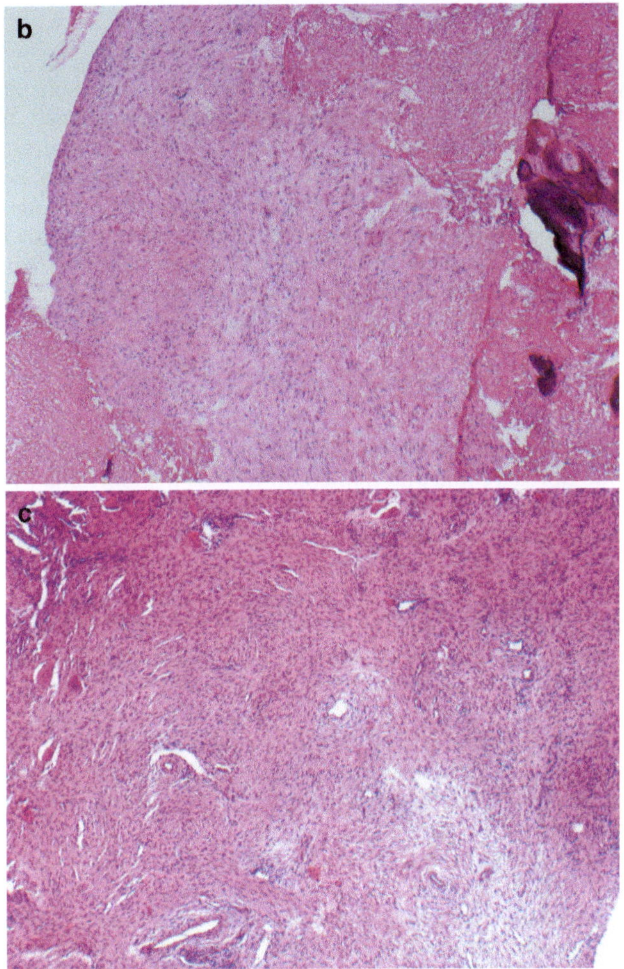

FIGURE 4.3 (continued)

FIGURE 4.3 Benign fibrous histiocytoma. A 29-year-old woman presented with significant leg pain. CT scan showed an expansile, lytic, and sclerotic lesion in the proximal diaphysis of the right fibula, with cortical thinning (**a**). Frozen sections showed loosely proliferative fibroblasts in a background of collagenized stroma, intermixed with small fragments of remodeled bone which may represent fracture callus (*right*) (**b**). Permanent sections showed a cellular spindle cell lesion with histologic features almost identical to those seen in a typical nonossifying fibroma (**c**). However, the age of patient, the presence of local pain, and the anatomic location of the lesion all point to a diagnosis of benign fibrous histiocytoma.

may breach the periostium and extend into the soft tissue. Histologically, the lesion is typically composed of dense, bland spindle cells in a background of richly collagenized matrix. The separation of desmoplastic fibroma from NOF/BFH may be difficult on histologic grounds even on permanent sections and especially in small curettage material. In these situations, the identification of its characteristic cytogenetic abnormalities (trisomies 8 and 20) and nuclear β-catenin accumulation, if present, can help reach the diagnosis of desmoplastic fibroma.

FIBROSARCOMA AND MALIGNANT FIBROUS HISTIOCYTOMA

Primary malignant fibrous/fibrohistiocytic lesions of bone include fibrosarcoma and malignant fibrous histiocytoma (MFH). Fibrosarcoma is far less common than previously thought, with many of those so labeled relabeled as monomorphic synovial sarcoma – thanks to advances in immunohistochemistry and molecular genetics. MFH is much more common than fibrosarcoma and may occur at any age, with a higher incidence in adults over 40 years. This tumor may arise de novo in bone but may also develop secondary to preexisting bone conditions such as radiation therapy for an unrelated malignancy or as a malignancy complicating Paget's disease or FD, or as the end product of "dedifferentiation" of a low-grade neoplasm. The aggressive behavior of these lesions is usually demonstrated by their destructive nature on imaging.

Histologically, fibrosarcoma is composed of a uniform population of spindled cells arranged in a fascicular or herringbone-like pattern, with a variable amount of collagenous matrix. The presence of readily discernable mitotic activity and hypercellularity in well-differentiated fibrosarcoma can distinguish it from desmoplastic fibroma. The lesion should be classified as myxofibrosarcoma in the presence of identifiable myxoid changes. Significant cytologic atypia, brisk mitotic activity, the presence of tumor giant cells, epitheloid type cells, and a storiform growth pattern are typically not present in fibrosarcoma and their presence would favor a diagnosis of MFH. Different histologic subtypes of MFH in bone (and soft tissue) have been described, including pleomorphic (Fig. 4.4), giant cell, and inflammatory. While MFH may have foci of osteoid and bone formation at the periphery of the lesion, these newly formed bony trabeculae are typically well organized and most typically represent periosteal reactive bone/fracture callus. Any unequivocal evidence of tumor cell-produced osteoid or bone should lead to a diagnosis of osteosarcoma (MFH-like; Fig. 4.5),

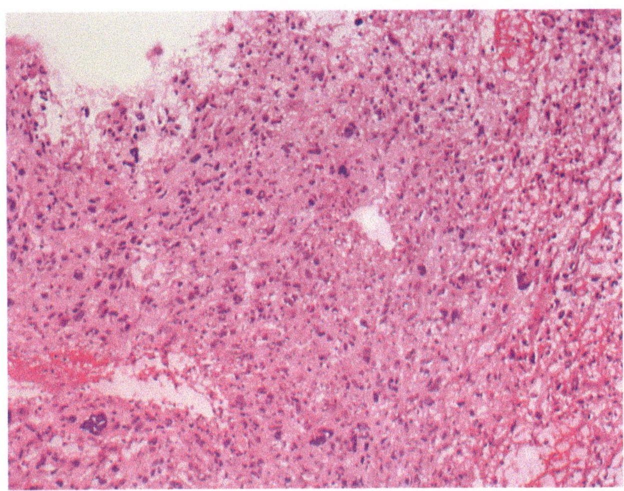

FIGURE 4.4 Malignant fibrous histiocytoma. This curettage specimen was from an aggressive lesion of femur in a 62-year-old man. Section showed a cellular neoplasm containing numerous large, bizarre cells, some with foamy cytoplasm. The tumor cells do not have apparent growth pattern or identifiable differentiation. No osteoid or new bone formation by tumor was present in either the frozen or the permanent sections. A diagnosis of malignant fibrous histiocytoma was rendered.

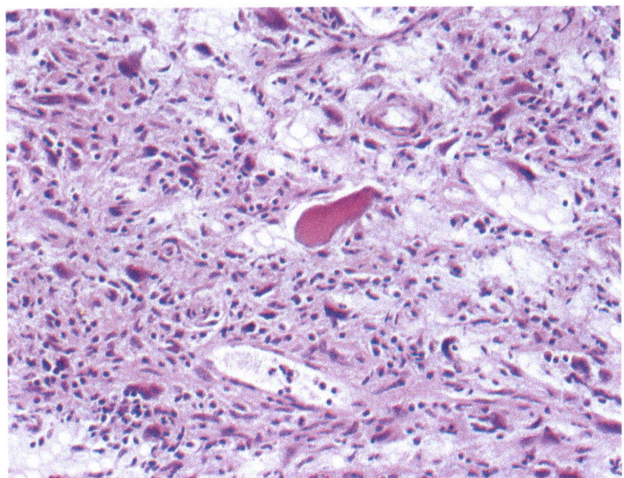

FIGURE 4.5 In contrast to the previous case, this is a section from a 3.0 cm lytic lesion in the distal third of tibia of a 60-year-old man. The section shows a highly pleomorphic sarcoma consisting of fibroblastic and fibrohistiocytic cells admixed with abundant bizarre multinucleated giant cells, mimicking a malignant fibrous histiocytoma. However, one can appreciate subtle but apparent tumor-produced bone matrix (*center*), thus rendering a diagnosis of osteosarcoma.

usually leading to neoadjuvant systemic chemotherapy prior to definitive surgical treatment. Given that such foci may be very subtle, a careful search of all sections is necessary.

FIBROUS DYSPLASIA

FD is a benign medullary fibro-osseous lesion, which is traditionally considered as a noninherited developmental disorder. However, recent studies have suggested that this entity is neoplastic in nature given the reproducible genetic abnormalities (activating mutations in the *GNAS1* gene and associated clonal chromosomal aberration). Nevertheless, FD may be a solitary (monostotic) lesion or of the polyostotic form. The latter is intimately associated with McCune–Albright syndrome (FD, endocrinopathy, and skin pigmentation) and Mazabraud syndrome (FD and intramuscular myxomas).

Although it can occur at any age, the majority of patients at first presentation of FD are younger than 30 years. The polyostotic form mostly presents in the first decade of life, while the monostotic form peaks in the late teens and early 20s. It may involve any bone, with long bones (femur and tibia), craniofacial bones, and ribs being most affected sites. The typical radiographic appearance is an expansile, lytic, or ground glass-like lesion with sharp margination in the metadiaphyseal region (if in long bones) (Fig. 4.6a).

The gross appearance of lesional tissue is usually dense and fibrous with a firm-gritty consistency. There may be cyst formation which may contain yellowish fluid. The classic microscopic findings include proliferating cytologically bland fibroblasts in a collagenous background, with bony trabeculae coursing irregularly throughout the lesion. These bone trabeculae, which are predominantly immature and woven in nature, are arranged in a haphazard manner and are commonly thin, curved or branching without osteoblastic rimming (Fig. 4.6b, c). Occasionally, the osteoid produced may take the form of rounded, cementum- or psammomatous-like bone, especially in craniofacial bones. Lipophages, multinucleated giant cells, and areas of cartilaginous differentiation (so-called "fibrocartilaginous dysplasia") may be present. No cytologic atypia is seen.

OSTEOFIBROUS DYSPLASIA

OFD has been also called *ossifying fibroma* and *Kempson–Campanacci's disease*. It is a benign fibro-osseous lesion that almost exclusively arises in the tibia, with or without involvement of the fibula. OFD predominantly occurs in children during the first two decades of life and typically involves the proximal or

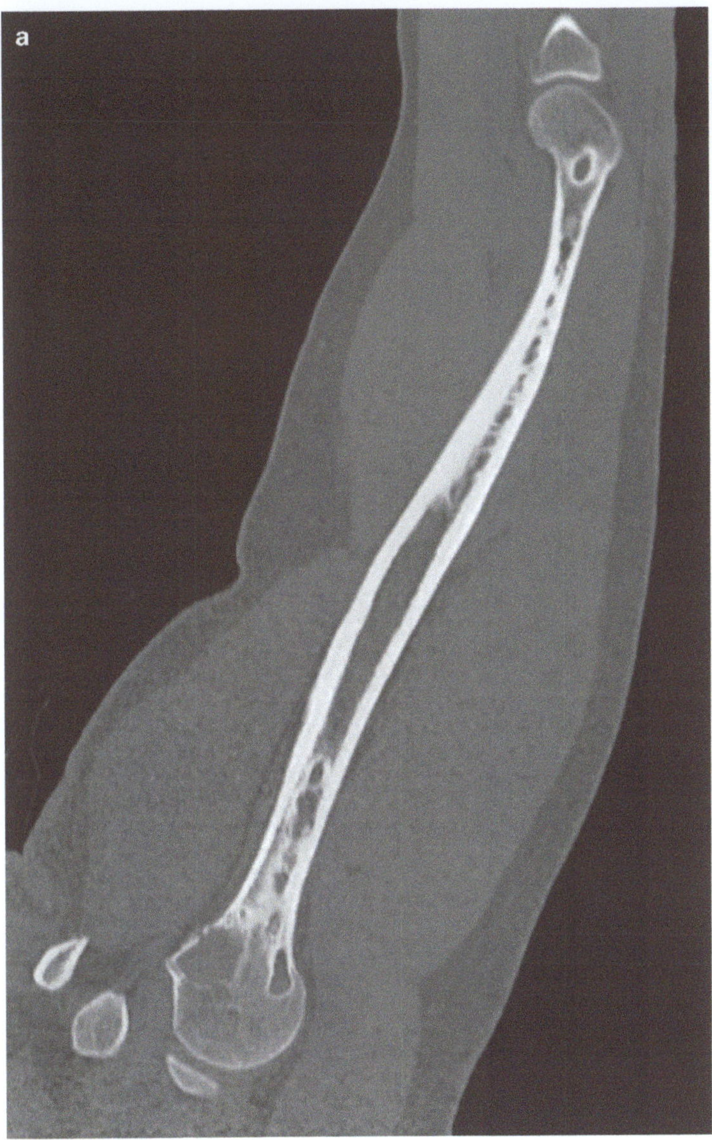

FIGURE 4.6 Fibrous dysplasia. This CT scan shows multiple well-demarcated lytic lesions in the proximal humerus, the largest involves the proximal humeral metadiaphysis with cortical breakthrough but no associated soft tissue mass or progressive periosteal reaction (**a**). Sections show a fibro-osseous lesion composed of irregularly shaped trabeculae of immature bone without rimming osteoblasts dispersed in a background of bland spindle cells (**b** and **c**). These findings are most consistent with fibrous dysplasia.

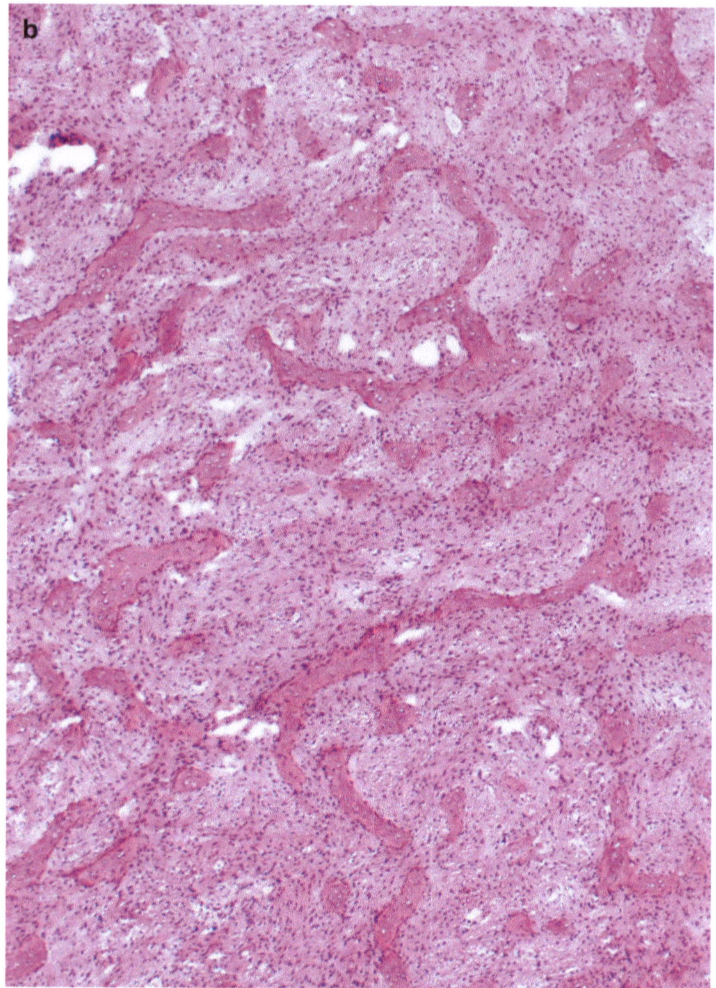

FIGURE 4.6 (continued)

middle-third of the tibial diaphysis. The majority of cases are self-limited and regress spontaneously after puberty. Thus, OFD represents a distinctly separate entity from FD.

On imaging, OFD most commonly affects the cortex anteriorly and presents as well-demarcated, multiloculated lytic expansion associated with a thin, sclerotic rim of cortex that separates the lesion from the medullary bone (Fig. 4.7a). Thus, the radiographic

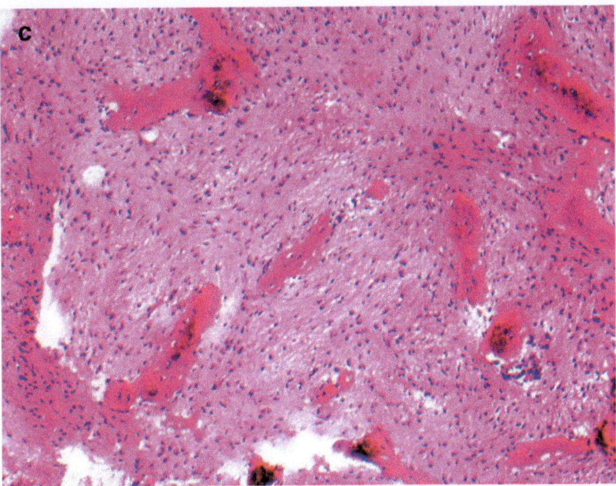

FIGURE 4.6 (continued)

appearance of OFD may closely mimic that of adamantinoma, a low-grade malignant biphasic tumor that involves particularly the anterior metadiaphysis of the tibia, although the latter typically affects patients in their 20s and 30s. A significant body of literature has emerged over the last few years, suggesting that the relationship between OFD and adamantinoma is, in fact, not coincidental and one may transform into the other over time. If the lesion involves the medullary cavity by extension, it may also resemble FD radiographically.

The histologic findings of OFD also resemble FD and are characterized by irregular fragments of woven bone trabeculae lying in variably cellular bland spindle cells with collagen production. In contrast to typical FD, the trabecular bone is rimmed, at least in part, by plump osteoblasts (Fig. 4.7b, c), which is also a differentiating feature from parosteal osteosarcoma (see Chap. 2). Osteoclasts may also be present. In contrast to adamantinoma, epithelial islands are absent. Other nonspecific findings include foamy histiocytes, hemorrhage, and cyst formation likely representing degenerative changes.

CENTRAL OSSIFYING FIBROMA

Central ossifying fibroma (COF) is a benign fibro-osseous neoplasm composed of cellular fibrous tissue admixed with varying amount of mineralized material, including bone and cementum, of

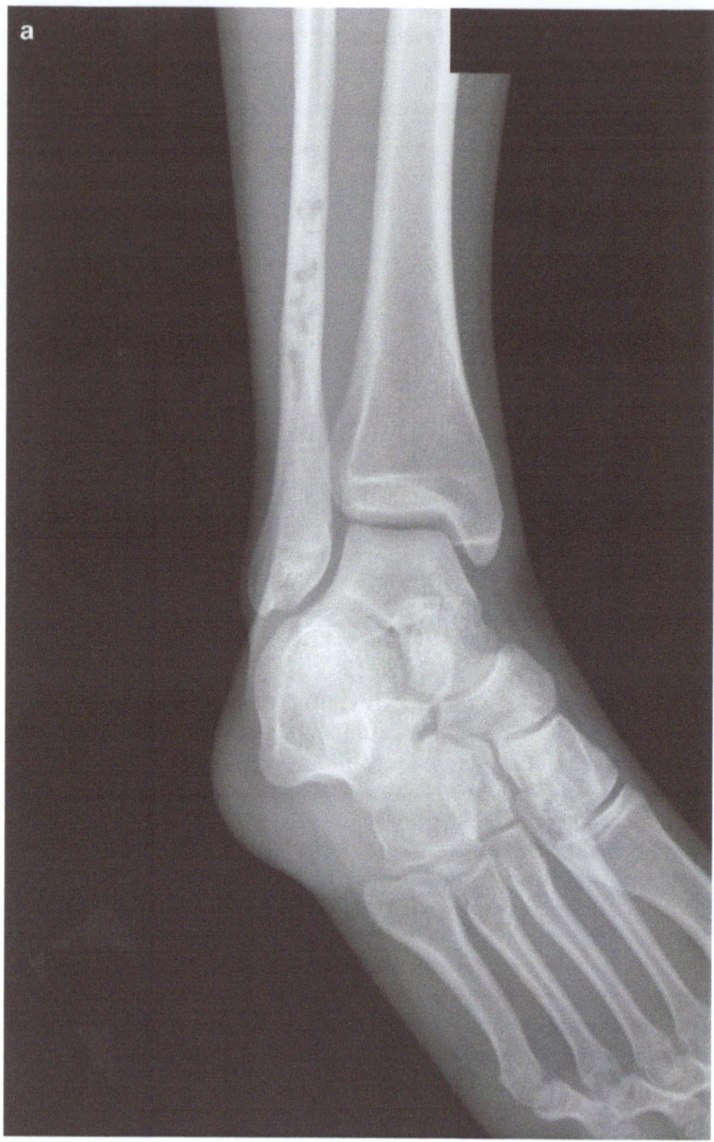

FIGURE 4.7 Osteofibrous dysplasia. This radiograph from an 11-year-old girl revealed multiple areas of radiolucency with surrounding osteosclerosis and a lack of a periosteal reaction in the cortical diaphysis of the right tibia (**a**). Frozen sections of this lesion show irregularly arranged bony trabeculae surrounded by a variably cellular fibroblastic proliferation (**b**). The bony trabeculae exhibit prominent osteoblastic rimming and increased osteoclast activity consistent with active remodeling (**c**). The spindle cells in the surrounding stroma display minimal cytologic atypia. This case demonstrates a perfect correlation between the radiologic and histopathologic findings and point to the diagnosis of osteofibrous dysplasia.

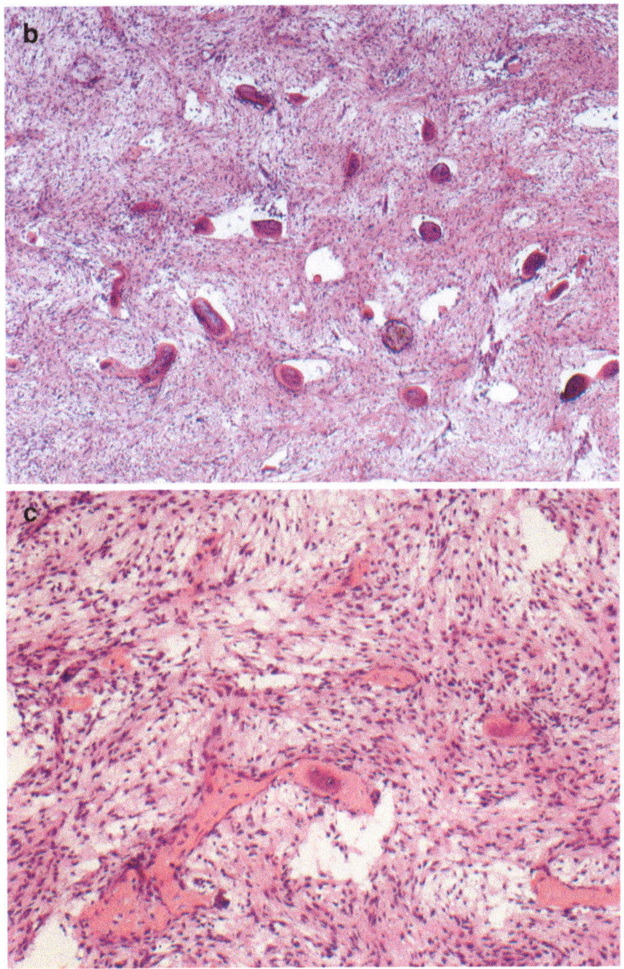

FIGURE 4.7 (continued)

varying appearance. COF most commonly occurs in the second to fourth decades of life, with a female predilection. It most frequently affects the mandible, especially the molar or posterior region.

COF is generally asymptomatic and diagnosed incidentally. Radiographs show a sharply demarcated or well-circumscribed lesion with smooth contours. The lesion may have radiodense as well as radiolucent areas, depending on the contributions of bone and soft tissue components.

Histologic sections of COF typically show randomly distributed bony spicules surrounded by variably cellular fibrous tissue. The mineralized trabeculae may consist of woven and/or lamellar bone and spherules of cementoid tissue (hence *cementifying fibroma* or *cemento-ossifying fibroma*). Psammomatoid OF, a unique variant of COF that mainly involves the paranasal sinuses, is characterized by a fibroblastic stroma containing bony spicules that resembles psammoma bodies (Fig. 4.8). The bony spicules of COF are typically rimmed by osteoblasts, but there may be mixed bands of cellular osteoid without osteoblastic rimming. The differential diagnosis of COF is primarily with FD. Distinction between these two lesions on histologic grounds only may be problematic. The most important distinguishing feature is the presence of demarcation and/or encapsulation in COF as opposed to the merging with its surroundings in FD.

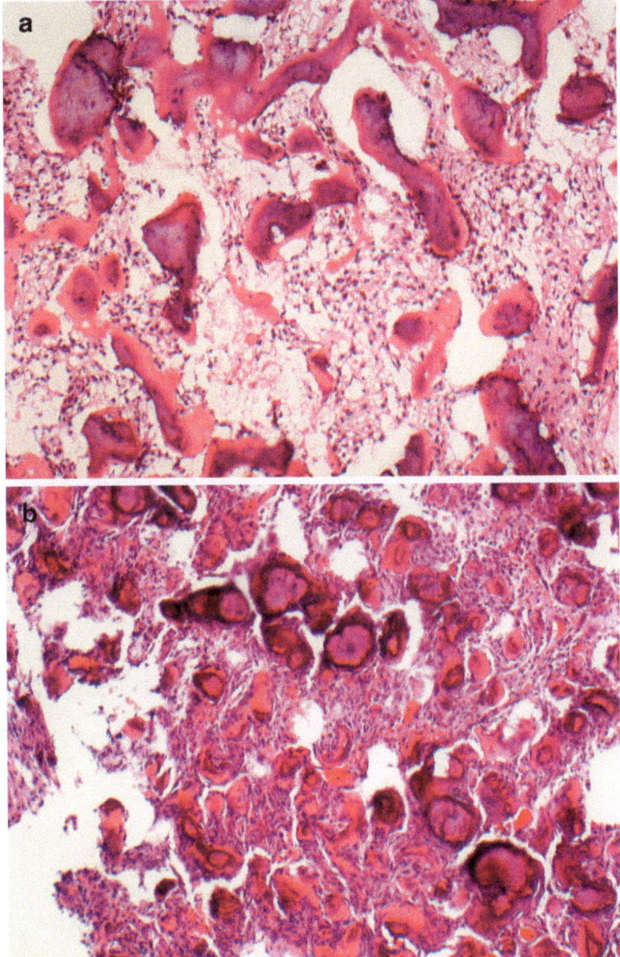

FIGURE 4.8 Central ossifying fibroma of the psammomatous type. This biopsy is from a 2.0 cm, well-demarcated, expansile mass involving the roof of the left orbit in a 64-year-old man. Frozen sections showed a fibro-osseous lesion consisting of irregularly shaped immature bony spicules admixed with variably cellular fibrous stroma (**a**). The permanent sections, however, revealed that the spicules were mostly spherical or curved resembling psammoma bodies (**b**). Taken together, the features are mostly consistent with central ossifying fibroma of the psammomatous type.

Chapter 5
Giant Cell-Rich Lesions

INTRODUCTION

Although almost all bone tumors contain giant cells, giant cell-rich lesions of bone encompass a number of entities in which the giant cells are an essential diagnostic component, chief among these are giant cell tumor (GCT) of bone, giant cell reparative granuloma (GCRG), and aneurysmal bone cyst (ABC). These lesions may have overlapping histomorphologic features, yet each possesses its own unique characteristics. Accordingly, clinical and radiologic input is necessary for definitive classification of these lesions.

In addition, a spectrum of other bony lesions may have on occasion prominent giant cell elements; these include principally giant cell-rich osteosarcoma, cherubism, and the so-called brown tumor of hyperparathyroidism. These lesions invariably have characteristic clinical and radiologic characteristics, i.e., aggressive growth in a non-epiphyseal location of a long bone (osteosarcoma), involvement of a particular anatomic site (the mandible in cherubism), unusual radiographic features (multifocal; subperiosteal bone resorption) and typical serum chemistries (brown tumor), and thus are frequently recognized prior to frozen section evaluation. Lastly, other primary tumors of bone may be mistaken for GCTs because the observer focuses on the osteoclast-like giant cells and ignores the other clinical, radiologic, and/or histomorphologic features; among these are chondroblastoma, nonossifying fibroma, and both benign and malignant fibrous histiocytomas.

GIANT CELL TUMOR OF BONE

GCT of bone was historically known as osteoclastoma. GCT is a locally aggressive neoplasm affecting principally young adults, with a slight female predominance. GCT is uncommon in

O. Hameed et al., *Frozen Section Library: Bone*, Frozen Section Library,
DOI 10.1007/978-1-4419-8376-3_5, © Springer Science+Business Media, LLC 2011

skeletally immature individuals and very rarely seen in children younger than 10 years.

Pain of variable severity is the most common and almost uniform presentation. GCT can affect any bone but typically involves the ends of long bones, principally around the knee (distal femur and proximal tibia). The sacrum is the most common site in the axial skeleton. Conventional radiographs of GCT in long bones usually show an eccentric, purely lytic, and expansile lesion, almost exclusively epiphyseal (or apophyseal) in location but may extend to adjacent metaphysis and articular cartilage (Fig. 5.1a). The margins may be well-defined with or without sclerosis, depending on the activity of the tumor. Mineralization within the lesion is distinctly uncommon. However, aggressive tumors may have ill-defined margins, cortical destruction, and soft-tissue extension, thus mimicking that of a biologically aggressive/malignant tumor.

The curetted fragments of tissue are typically soft and friable. The characteristic histopathological appearance is of evenly distributed, numerous osteoclast-like multinucleated giant cells (often containing 50–100 nuclei; Fig. 5.1b, c) in a background of sheets of uniform, oval to polygonal mononuclear stromal cells which resemble macrophages. It is now generally accepted that these mononuclear cells represent the neoplastic component. At higher magnification, the giant cell nuclei are similar to the nuclei of the neoplastic mononuclear cells in that they have regular outlines with open chromatin and small nucleoli. The cytoplasm is ill defined (Fig. 5.2a, b). In select areas, the mononuclear cells can be more spindle-shaped and may even be arranged in a storiform growth pattern (Fig. 5.3). Collections of foam (xanthoma) cells may also be present. This phenomenon, when dominating the histologic appearance, may lead to a mistaken diagnosis of a benign fibrous histiocytoma (see Chap. 4). The stroma is typically rich in vasculature (but not usually to the same degree as seen in GCRG) and intravascular invasion in the form of "plugs of tumor cells" is frequently seen (Fig. 5.4). Mitotic figures may be abundant, but atypical mitoses are not seen and their presence should point to an alternative diagnosis of a giant cell-rich sarcoma. There should be no cytologic atypia in a typical GCT. The tumor typically lacks extensive matrix production; however, in our experience, small foci of osteoid and woven bone are invariably present, especially in lesions associated with pathologic fracture, at the periphery or at the leading edges of a soft tissue recurrence resulting in a characteristic "egg-shell" appearance on conventional radiographs. This is often difficult to appreciate on frozen sectioning because the curettings have no preserved geographic relationship with the adjacent bone or soft tissue structures.

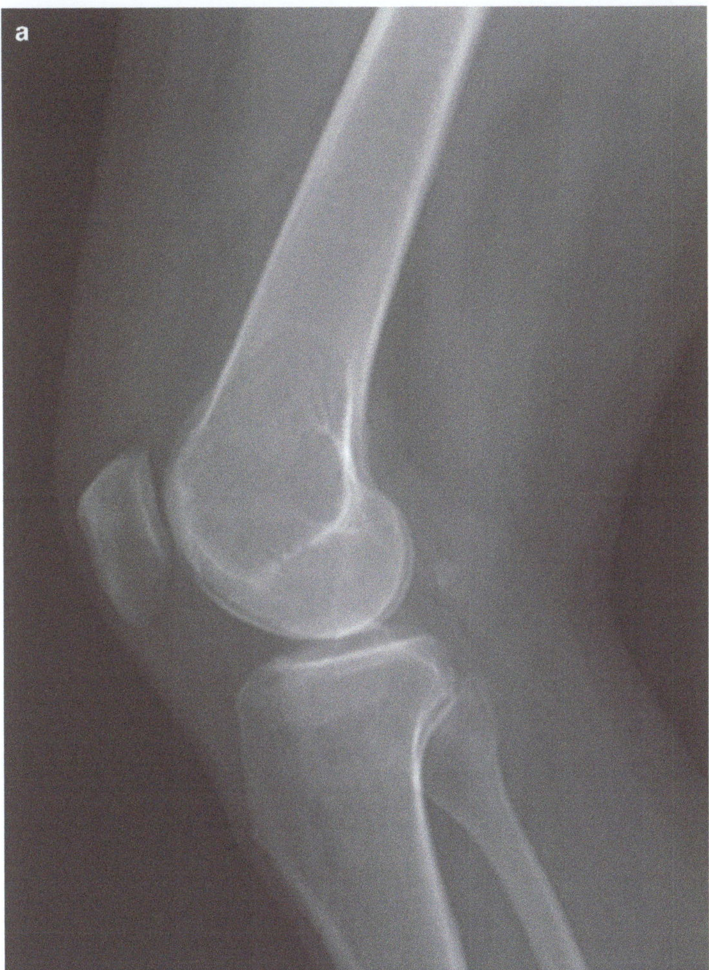

FIGURE 5.1 Giant cell tumor of bone. The conventional radiograph of a 46-year-old woman reveals a large lucent lesion occupying the right medial femoral condyle (**a**). The lesion extends distally to the articular surface and proximally into the diametaphyseal region. The lesion is sharply marginated with a minimal periosteal reaction. There are no lesional contents. Frozen sections from the lucent region displayed numerous, large osteoclast-type multinucleated giant cells which lie uniformly in a syncytium of round to oval mononuclear cells (**b**). There are areas suggestive of cyst formation but these may also represent freezing artifact. At intermediate magnification, the mononuclear cells as well as the multinucleated giant cells have eosinophilic cytoplasm and indistinct cell borders, with vesicular nuclei and small nucleoli. The nuclei of mononuclear cells and those of the multinucleated cells are similar in appearance (**c**). The overall findings are typical for a giant cell tumor with excellent radiologic–pathologic correlation.

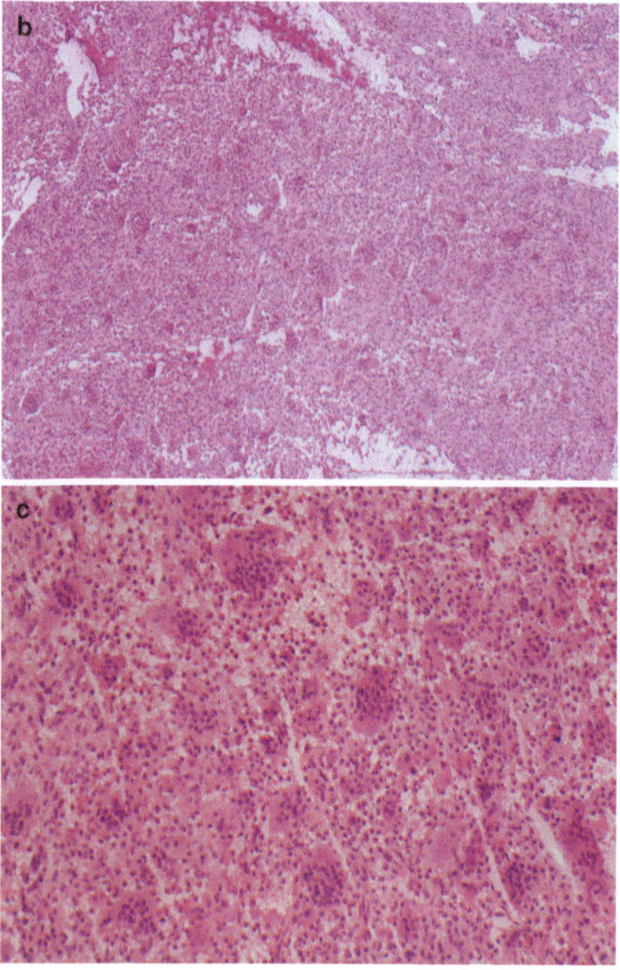

FIGURE 5.1 (continued)

When present, the new bone formation has the appearance of a reactive process with prominent osteoblastic rimming of the bony trabeculae, similar to that commonly seen in an ABC. Other common but nonspecific findings include focal necrosis, hemorrhage, and hemosiderin deposition.

While most GCTs have characteristic clinical, radiologic, and histopathologic manifestations allowing for a straightforward diagnosis, a lesion that fulfills all the clinical and radiologic

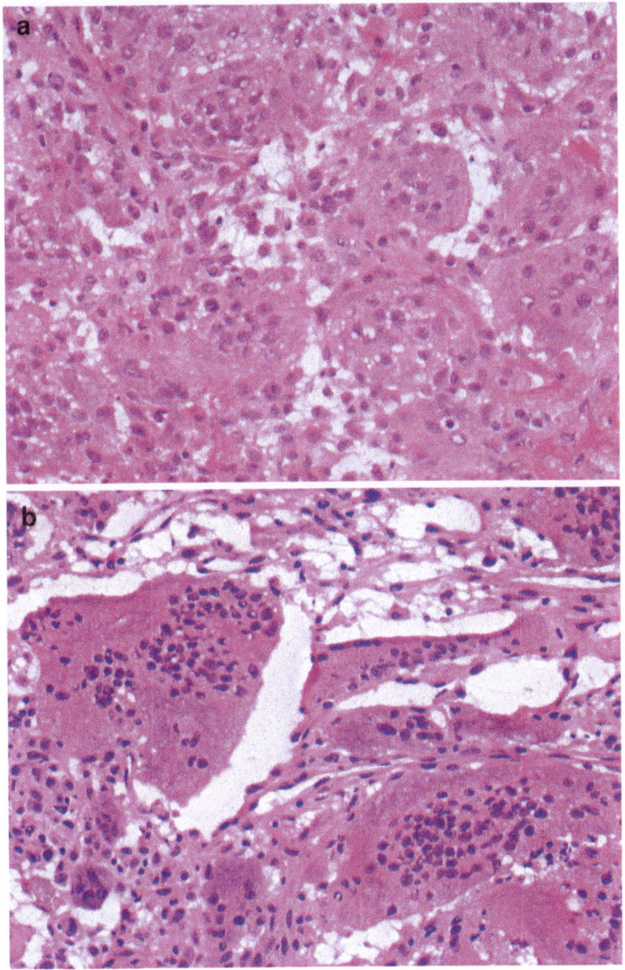

FIGURE 5.2 High power views (**a** and **b**) of a giant cell tumor of bone. The giant cells may be very large and contain 50–100 nuclei (**b**).

features of a GCT should be regarded as a GCT even if there is only a minimal typical GCT component histologically, especially during intraoperative consultation with limited material from curettage specimens. On the other hand, as alluded to above, virtually any tumor of bone may contain variable numbers of multinucleated giant cells. However, both the presence of large, confluent, osteoclast-like, multinucleated giant cells and the

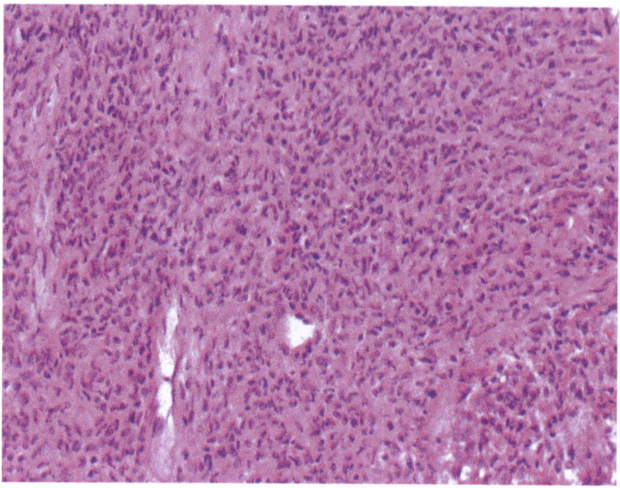

FIGURE 5.3 Giant cell tumor of bone with prominent spindled cells. These areas are often devoid of giant cells and may resemble a benign fibrous histiocytoma.

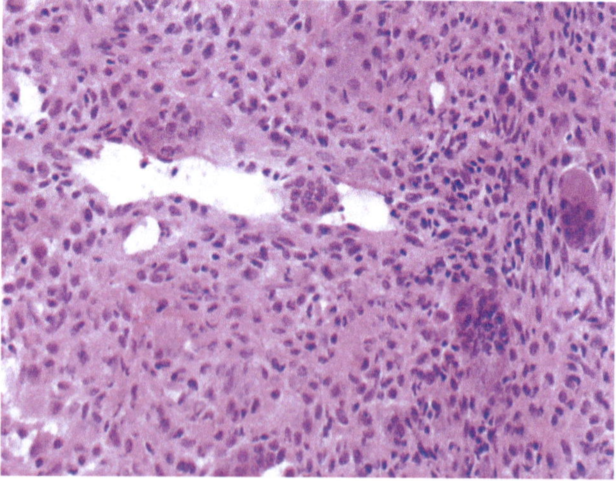

FIGURE 5.4 Giant cell tumor of bone with intravascular invasion in the form of "plugs of tumor cells."

cytologic resemblance of giant cell nuclei to ovoid or spindled mononuclear cell nuclei are typically absent in lesions other than GCT such as ABC, chondroblastoma, GCRG, and malignant bone lesions with prominent giant cells.

ANEURYSMAL BONE CYST AND OTHER MIMICS

Primary ABC is a benign but locally aggressive cystic lesion that commonly affects patients in the first two decades of life. It usually arises in the metaphysis of long bones but less frequently involves the vertebrae, characteristically situated in the dorsal elements.

Primary ABC typically presents as a lytic, eccentric, expansile mass with well-defined margins on conventional radiographs. CT and MRI studies frequently show internal septa and characteristic fluid–fluid levels (Fig. 5.5a). Microscopically, pure ABC is

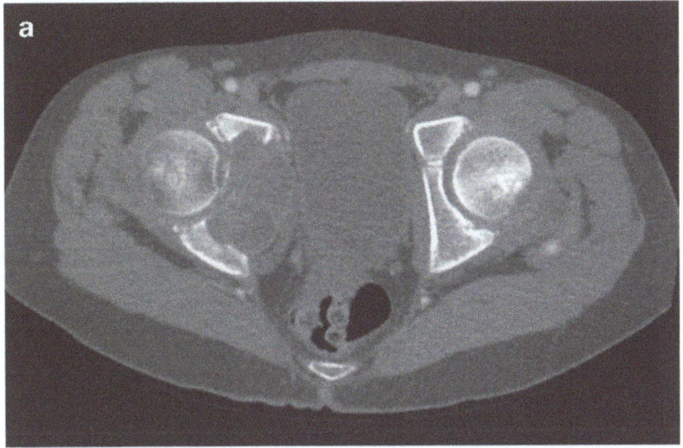

FIGURE 5.5 Primary aneurysmal bone cyst. A 15-year-old boy presented with increasing pain involving his right hip. CT scan revealed a well-defined, heterogeneous, expansile lytic lesion in his right acetabulum (**a**). The mass was predominantly hypodense with internal septa and multiple fluid levels. This appearance is mostly consistent with an aneurysmal bone cyst. Although very unlikely, a telangiectatic osteosarcoma could not be entirely excluded. Frozen sections showed a hemorrhagic lesion, of which the solid component was composed of a fibrotic cyst wall devoid of apparent lining (**b**). The cellular compartments included spindled fibroblasts, osteoclast-type multinucleated giant cells, and hemosiderin (**b**). In addition, thin strands of reactive woven bone formation were present along the cyst wall and within the fibrotic stroma (**c** and **d**). The newly formed bone is rimmed by flat, but more commonly plumped or plasmacytoid osteoblasts (**d**). No significant cytologic atypia or other complicating lesional tissue was found. Thus, a diagnosis of primary aneurysmal bone cyst was rendered.

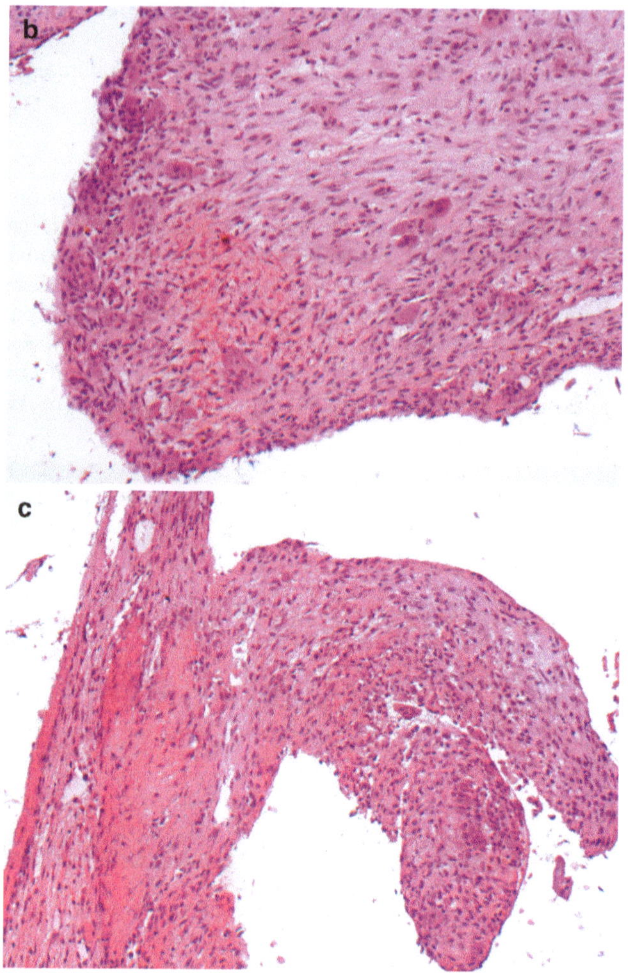

FIGURE 5.5   (continued)

composed of blood-filled, variably sized cystic spaces separated by fibrous septa, which contain predominantly proliferative fibroblasts, and scattered osteoclast-like multinucleated giant cells (Fig. 5.5b). Reactive new bone formation, typically in the form of thin strands, is almost invariably present, commonly along the cyst wall (Fig. 5.5c, d). However, ABC may also arise secondarily in association with other benign or malignant bone tumors.

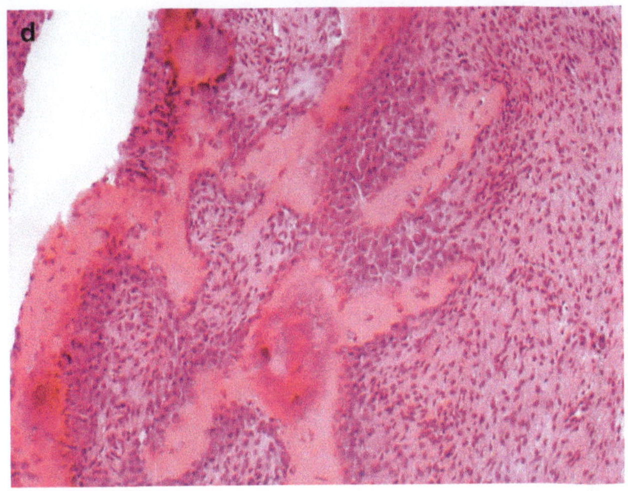

FIGURE 5.5 (continued)

In fact, secondary ABC is not uncommonly associated with a GCT (Fig. 5.6). While CT and MRI may show evidence of an underlying primary lesion in such circumstances, a lesion with the histologic appearance of an ABC but extending to the end of a long bone should prompt the pathologist to conduct a thorough search for even small foci of typical GCT.

Chondroblastoma, like GCT, classically also occurs in epiphysis of long bones but typically affects skeletally immature patients. The important histological features to distinguish GCT from a chondroblastoma are lack of chondroid differentiation, no chicken wire matrix, and uniformly distributed giant cells that are larger and contain more numerous nuclei than typically appreciated in chondroblastoma (see Chap. 3).

As noted previously, malignant bone tumors may also contain giant cell elements. The nature of malignancy may be appreciated by the aggressive growth and the histologic appearance (i.e., the degree of cellular atypia, atypical mitotic figures, and necrosis). Most of these lesions represent osteosarcoma (Fig. 5.7), malignant fibrous histiocytoma, or sarcoma with a dedifferentiated component (Fig. 5.8) resembling GCT. It should be noted, however, that malignancy in GCT (also known as malignant GCT) is either a high-grade sarcoma arising in a GCT (primary) or at the site of previously documented GCT (secondary). While a de novo

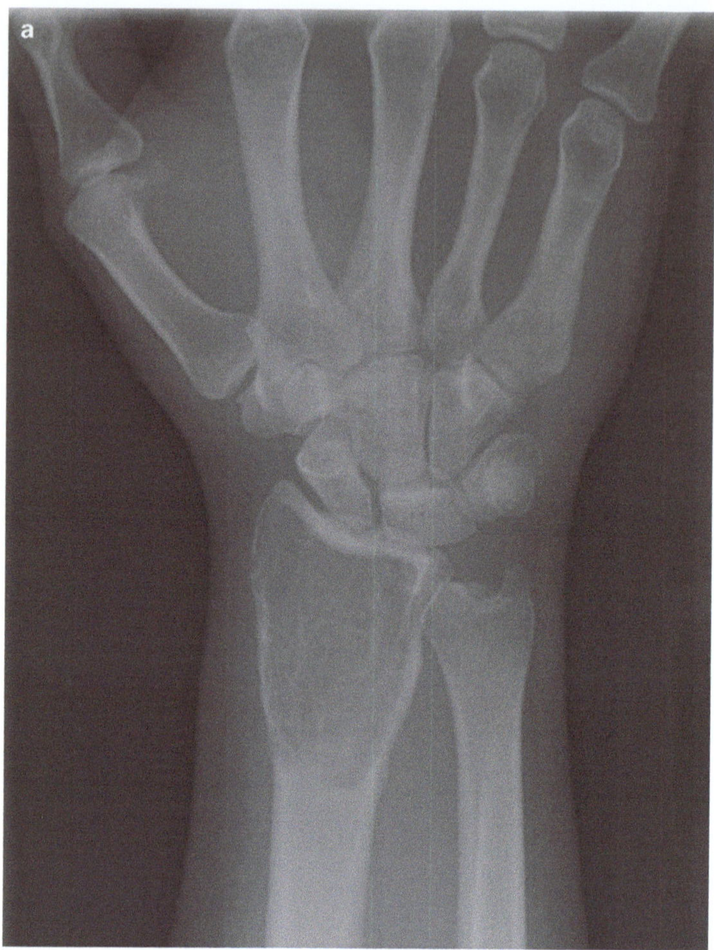

FIGURE 5.6 Secondary aneurysmal bone cyst. A 37-year-old man presented with local pain. Conventional imaging shows an expanded lytic lesion extending to the subarticular portion of the right distal radius with sharp, nonsclerotic margins (**a**). There is no obvious cortical breakthrough or periosteal reaction. There are internal septations but no matrix is present. The radiological differential diagnosis includes giant cell tumor and aneurysmal bone cyst. Alternatively, this may also represent a giant cell tumor with a secondary aneurysmal bone cyst. Upon frozen sectioning the lesion is that of a giant cell tumor which consists, in most areas, of confluent osteoclast-like, multinucleated giant cells in a background of mononuclear cells (**b**, *right upper*, and **c**). However, nonendothelium-lined cyst spaces consisting of lakes of blood are also present. Fibroblastic proliferation and formation of osteoid and bone trabeculae are seen in areas (**b**, *center*, **d**, *upper right* and **e**). The findings are mostly consistent with a giant cell tumor with secondary aneurysmal bone cyst formation which was confirmed on permanent sections.

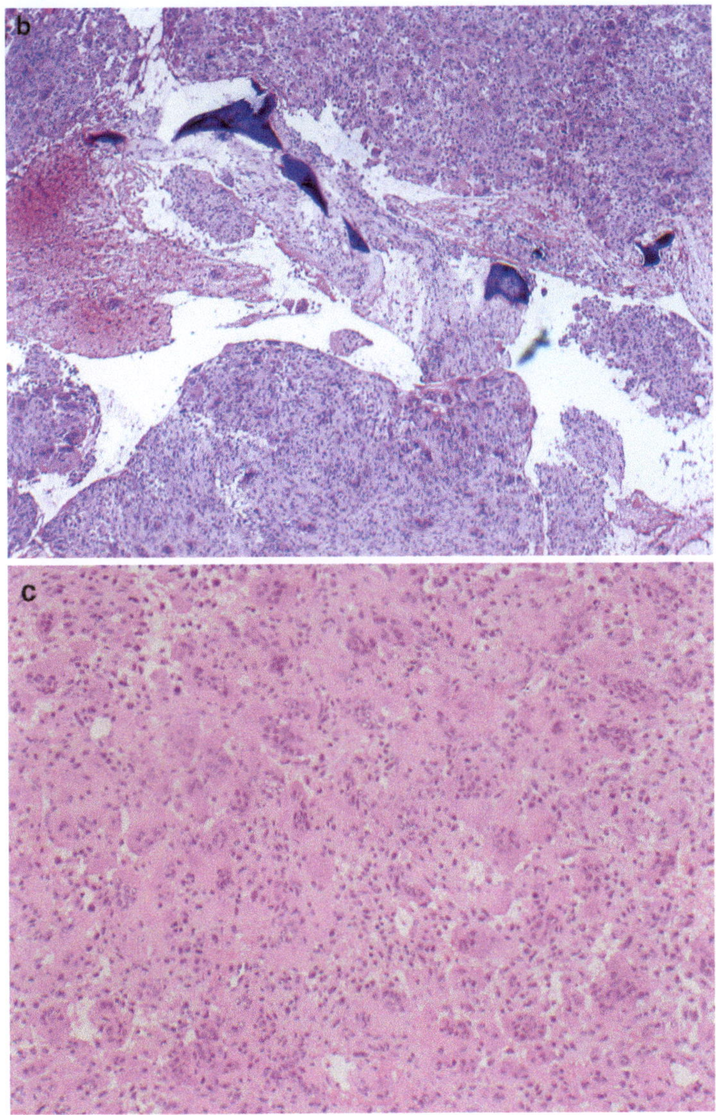

FIGURE 5.6 (continued)

malignant GCT may have the same radiographic appearance as a benign GCT, there are areas of conventional GCT and concurrent high-grade spindle-cell sarcoma with an abrupt transition in dedifferentiated forms. A secondary malignant GCT typically arises in the same location several years after a previous GCT, usually following radiation therapy.

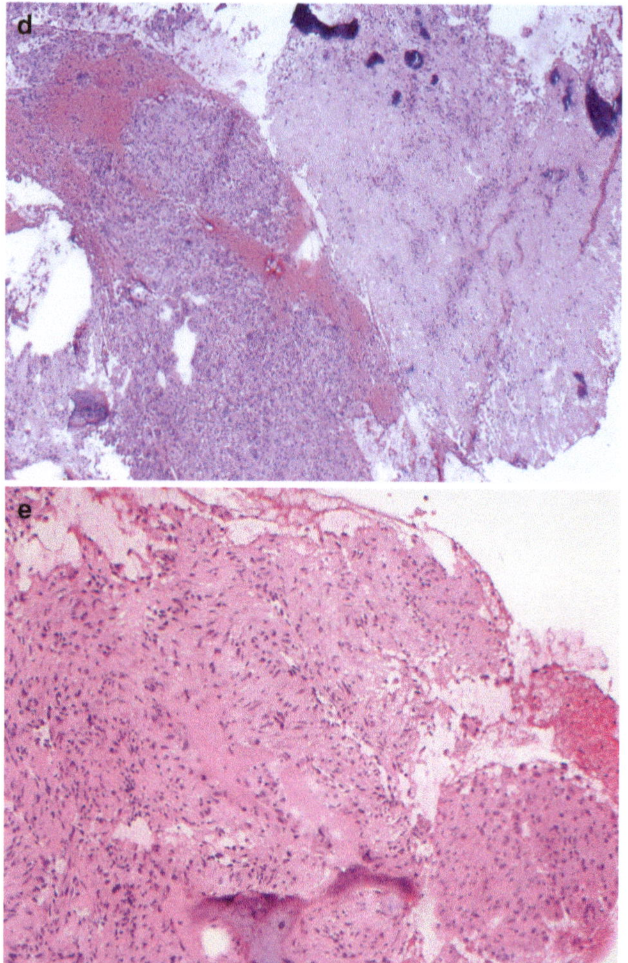

FIGURE 5.6 (continued)

GIANT CELL REPARATIVE GRANULOMA

GCRG was first described as a nonneoplastic fibrous lesion with scattered osteoclast-like multinucleated giant cells of gnathic bones in children and young adults. Thereafter, the concept of GCRG of extragnathic sites (also known as giant cell reaction) has been widely recognized. Meanwhile, given the significant histopathologic overlap, GCRG of extragnathic sites has been

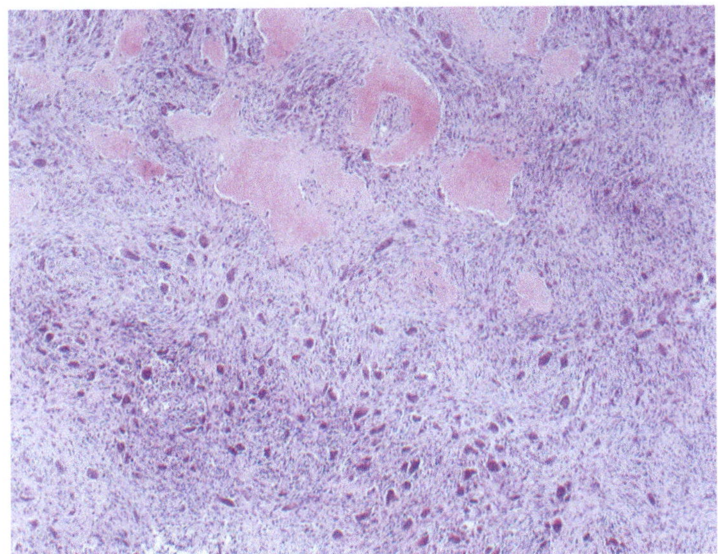

FIGURE 5.7 Giant cell-rich osteosarcoma. Note that without the nested giant cell component, the tumor is otherwise a typical conventional osteosarcoma, with tumor osteoid filling the upper half of the section. Although many giant cell-rich osteosarcomas are similar to telangiectatic osteosarcomas, this example has more of a fibroblastic appearance.

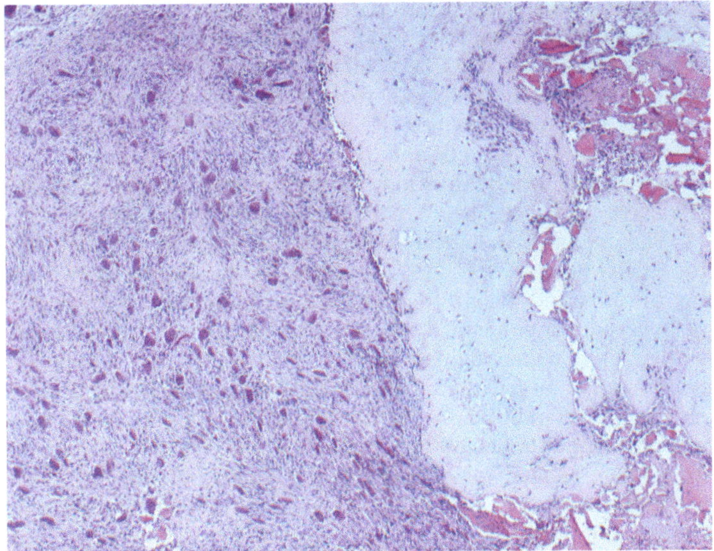

FIGURE 5.8 The permanent section of a dedifferentiated chondrosarcoma. Note the abrupt transition of a well-differentiated chondrosarcoma from its dedifferentiated component resembling giant cell tumor of bone.

merged with the entity "solid variant of aneurysmal bone cyst (solid ABC)" by many practitioners.

Characteristic radiographic features occurring in the GCRG of maxilla and mandible are the presence of a round or oval lucency with fine trabeculations and distinct borders. Extragnathic GCRGs frequently occur in the small bones of the hands and feet and very rarely in long tubular bones and vertebrae. On imaging, lesions may be intramedullary or rarely surface based and can be metaphyseal or diaphyseal, but do not cross the open growth plate in skeletally immature patients. The most characteristic radiologic features are purely lytic and expansile lesions with sharp margination, regardless of location. Soft tissue extension beyond the cortex is uncommon but may be occasionally seen. On MRI, fluid–fluid levels among solid components are often seen within the lesion, which correspond to small cysts filled with blood akin to secondary ABCs.

The curetted fragments of bone are tan or reddish brown, friable, gritty tissues. Low-power microscopic examination typically reveals a moderately to highly cellular spindle-cell proliferation in the background of vascular-rich fibrous stroma that often contains varying amount of collagen fibers. Numerous osteoclast-like multinucleated giant cells are unevenly distributed throughout the lesion and tend to be arranged in a vaguely clustered fashion (Fig. 5.9a). Microscopic evidence of hemorrhagic cyst formation reminiscent of an ABC, as well as hemosiderin deposition, is frequently seen. Newly formed reactive osteoid or bone trabeculae rimmed by osteoblasts are an extremely common finding. The spindled fibroblastic cells and the giant cells lack cytologic atypia. Occasional mitotic figures may be present but not atypical forms (Fig. 5.9b, c).

The major histological differential diagnostic consideration for GCRG includes ABC, GCT, fibrohistiocytic lesions (nonossifying fibroma and benign fibrous histiocytoma), and brown tumor of hyperparathyroidism. The cellular components of an ABC are similar, if not identical, to a GCRG. However, ABC is typically composed of larger blood-filled cysts (lakes of blood) and has a characteristic radiographic presentation. A GCT may rarely have a prominent spindle-cell component. However, GCTs are almost exclusively located in an epiphyseal region, and the giant cells are typically larger, confluent, and evenly arranged. Nonossifying fibroma and benign fibrous histiocytoma do not typically have reactive new bone formation within the lesion, and the giant cells

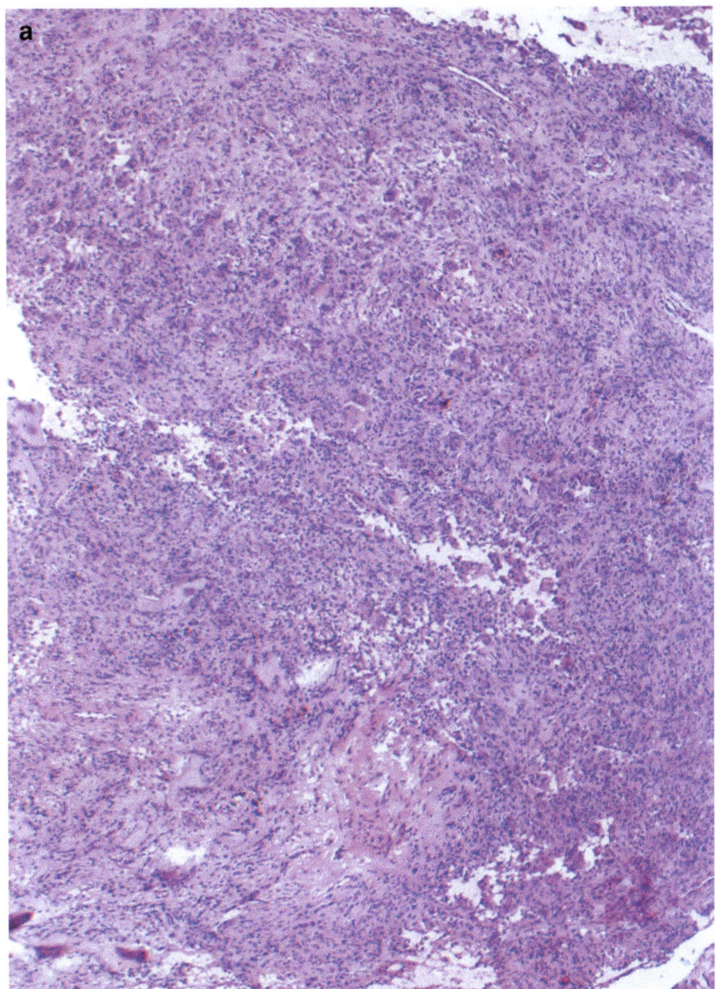

FIGURE 5.9 Giant cell reparative granuloma. A 50-year-old man presented with back pain. An MRI demonstrated a densely enhancing mass involving the L4 vertebral body, displacing adjacent paravertebral structures. Frozen sections reveal a densely cellular lesion consisting of spindled mononuclear cells and abundant, randomly distributed osteoclast-like multinucleated giant cells in a focally hyalinized stroma with intermixed hemosiderin deposition (**a**). At higher magnification, one can appreciate the cellular details of the mononuclear stromal cells and the giant cells which, as seen in aneurysmal bone cyst, lack significant cytologic atypia (**b** and **c**). However, cavernous spaces filled with lakes of blood, a feature characteristic of aneurysmal bone cyst, are not present. The fibrous stroma is highly vascularized and composed of reactive osteoid and new bone formation (**b** and **c**). Thus, the features are those of a typical giant cell reparative granuloma.

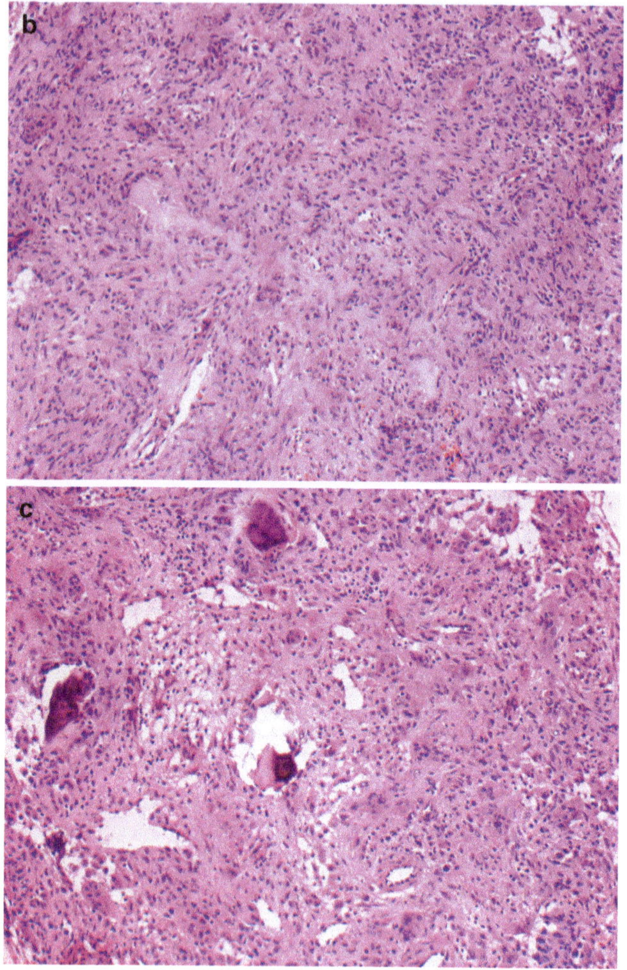

Figure 5.9 (continued)

are usually smaller and randomly distributed (see Chap. 4). Brown tumor is almost indistinguishable microscopically from a GCRG and historically has always been in the differential diagnosis, but as this entity has become extremely uncommon or recognized presurgically, it rarely causes a clinical problem. If in doubt, a comment with a recommendation for clinical laboratory testing is appropriate.

Chapter 6
Small/Round Cell Lesions

INTRODUCTION

Lesions considered in this chapter include traditional "small blue round cell" neoplasms, specifically Ewing sarcoma/primitive neuroectodermal tumor (ES/PNET) and lymphomas, solitary plasmacytoma/multiple myeloma, and other lesions that tend to be composed of a mixed population of rounded cells without epithelial differentiation or significant extracellular matrix deposition. These latter lesions include osteomyelitis and Langerhans cell histiocytosis (LCH). As discussed earlier, however, there are other lesions that can be composed predominantly of small round cells, such as small cell osteosarcoma (Chap. 2), which may also need to be considered in the differential diagnosis.

EWING SARCOMA/PRIMITIVE NEUROECTODERMAL TUMOR

Although ES/PNET has been described at various ages, most patients present before their 20th birthday with pain and a mass lesion. The classic location for this neoplasm is the diaphyses of long bones, but it may also arise in the axial bones such as the pelvis and ribs (as well as in soft tissues and other organs). Patients may also present with fever and leukocytosis suggesting an infectious picture, which is important to remember especially since osteomyelitis often has overlapping clinical and radiological findings (see below). Radiologically, a destructive permeative lesion is usually evident within the diaphysis of a long bone (Fig. 6.1) often with an overlying multilayered but discontinuous "onion-skin" periosteal reaction. Occasionally, there is a large soft tissue mass with no obvious bone destruction on the conventional radiographs,

O. Hameed et al., *Frozen Section Library: Bone*, Frozen Section Library,
DOI 10.1007/978-1-4419-8376-3_6, © Springer Science+Business Media, LLC 2011

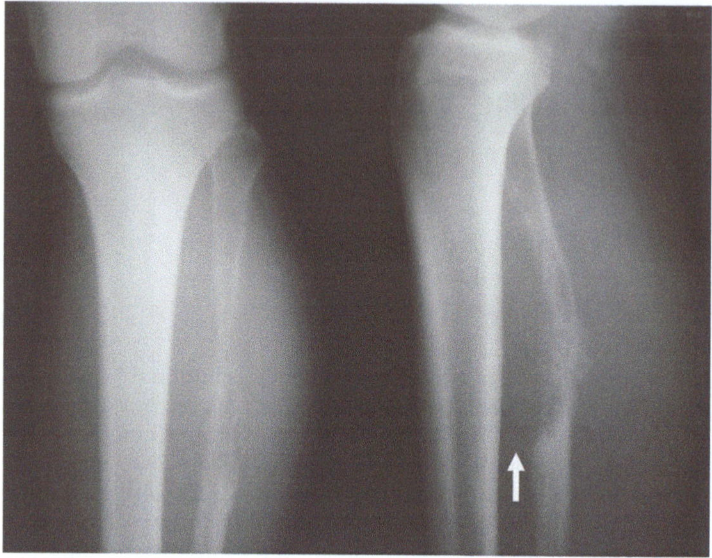

FIGURE 6.1 Ewing sarcoma involving the diaphysis of the fibula. Notice the marked cortical destruction and the elevated periosteum (*arrow*) (image courtesy of Mark J. Kransdorf, Mayo Clinic, Jacksonville, FL).

but the intraosseous component becomes evident on a CT scan or MRI. Histologically, Ewing sarcoma is composed of sheets of small-rounded cells, with amphophilic cytoplasm and uniform hyperchromatic nuclei (Fig. 6.2). Evidence of neuroectodermal differentiation may be identified even on frozen section evaluation as extracellular eosinophilic neuropil-like structures or Homer-Wright rosettes, which are composed of groups of tumor cells that surround a central core of the eosinophilic extracellular material. If these are very prominent, metastatic neuroblastoma needs to be eliminated as a diagnostic possibility. The histological differential diagnosis of ES/PNET in this age group would also include lymphoma (see below) as well as other small round cell tumors of childhood that have metastasized to bone, most principally rhabdomyosarcoma.

LYMPHOMA

Most bone lymphomas are secondary to disease elsewhere, but primary bone lymphomas most certainly occur. The majority of primary bone lymphomas, and those that secondarily involve the bone as tumorous masses, are diffuse large B-cell lymphomas and a few other high-grade tumors, whereas most lower-grade lymphomas and leukemias present with diffuse marrow involvement rather

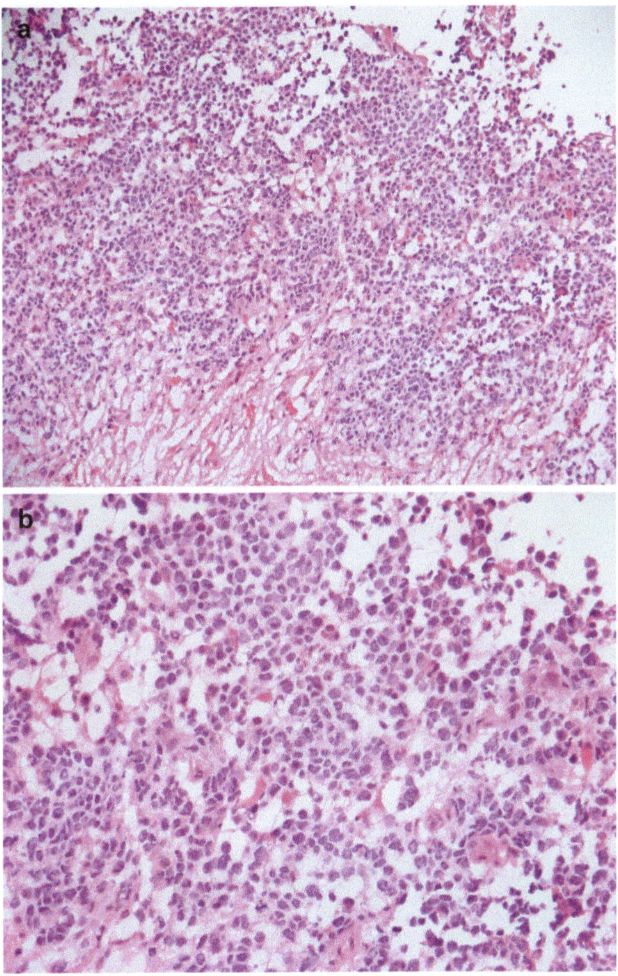

FIGURE 6.2 An example of Ewing sarcoma (**a**, **b**) in which sheets of small round blue cells are evident on frozen section. Even on high power (**b**), it is very difficult to distinguish this from hematopoietic neoplasms.

than mass lesions. Radiologically, lymphomas usually present as radiolucent lesions (Fig. 6.3), sometimes disproportionately destructive when compared with the patient's clinical symptoms. The histological findings on frozen section evaluation are similar to those seen in extraskeletal lymphomas and are characterized by the presence of sheets of noncohesive, rounded, hyperchromatic cells, usually with some (but minimal) pleomorphism (Fig. 6.4).

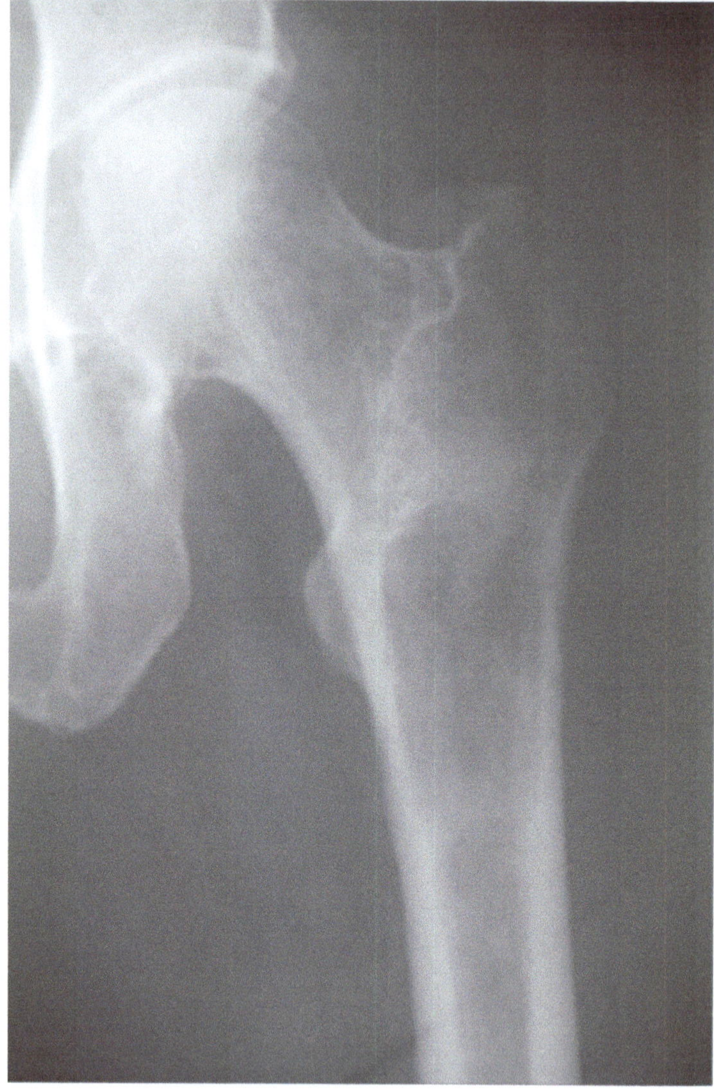

FIGURE 6.3 On conventional radiographs, lymphomas usually appear as destructive osteolytic lesions without a surrounding sclerotic rim, as seen in the subtrochanteric area of this femur (image courtesy of Dr. Michael J. Klein, Hospital for Special Surgery, New York, NY).

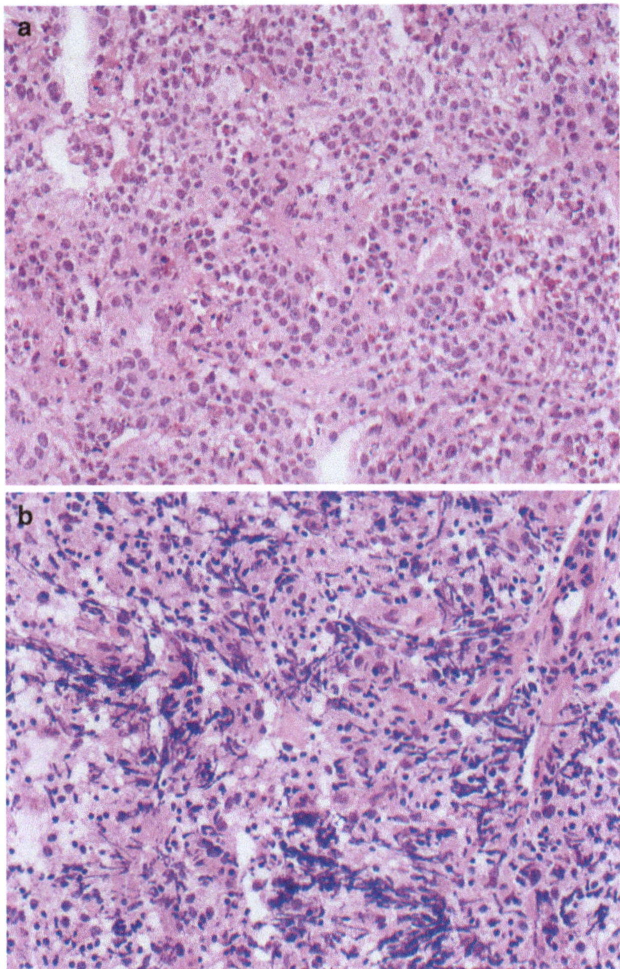

FIGURE 6.4 Bone lymphomas evaluated by frozen section. The first example (**a**) is composed of sheets of large cells having indistinct cytoplasmic borders and rounded nuclei with occasionally prominent nucleoli. Prominent apoptosis is present. A more polymorphic population is evident in the second case (**b**) where significant nuclear crushing is also present. Although the neoplasm is less cellular in the third case (**c**) with smaller tumor cells and is potentially more suggestive of an inflammatory process (osteomyelitis), the prominent hyperchromasia present (even at this magnification) helps to point toward the diagnosis of lymphoma.

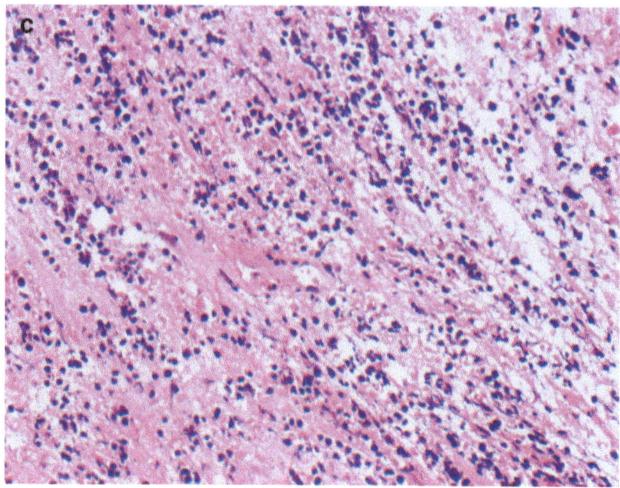

FIGURE 6.4 (continued)

The latter is useful in distinguishing this lesion from its mimickers including Ewing sarcoma and small cell carcinoma, which tend to have more monotonous cytology (and more finely dispersed chromatin), and poorly differentiated carcinomas, which tend to be more pleomorphic. Of note, a touch preparation of the submitted material can be very useful in distinguishing between these lesions and from plasma cell lesions (see below).

SOLITARY PLASMACYTOMA AND MULTIPLE MYELOMA

Despite the quite variable presentation of myeloma, it is frequently in the differential diagnosis on frozen sections because it accounts for a large percentage of small, blue, round cell tumors arising primarily in the bone of adults (as opposed to infants [neuroblastoma, rhabdomyosarcoma, and LCH], teenagers [ES/PNET], or young adults [lymphoma, small cell osteosarcoma]). Involvement of the skeletal system is usually manifested by bone pain and/or pathological fractures. Radiologically, plasmacytoma and the lesions of multiple myeloma are lytic, well-demarcated and without a rim of sclerotic bone (Fig. 6.5); however, multiple myeloma may also present with "generalized osteoporosis" without any detectable foci of discrete bone destruction. As one would expect, solitary plasmacytoma and bone lesions of multiple myeloma are histologically composed of plasma cells and their precursors at

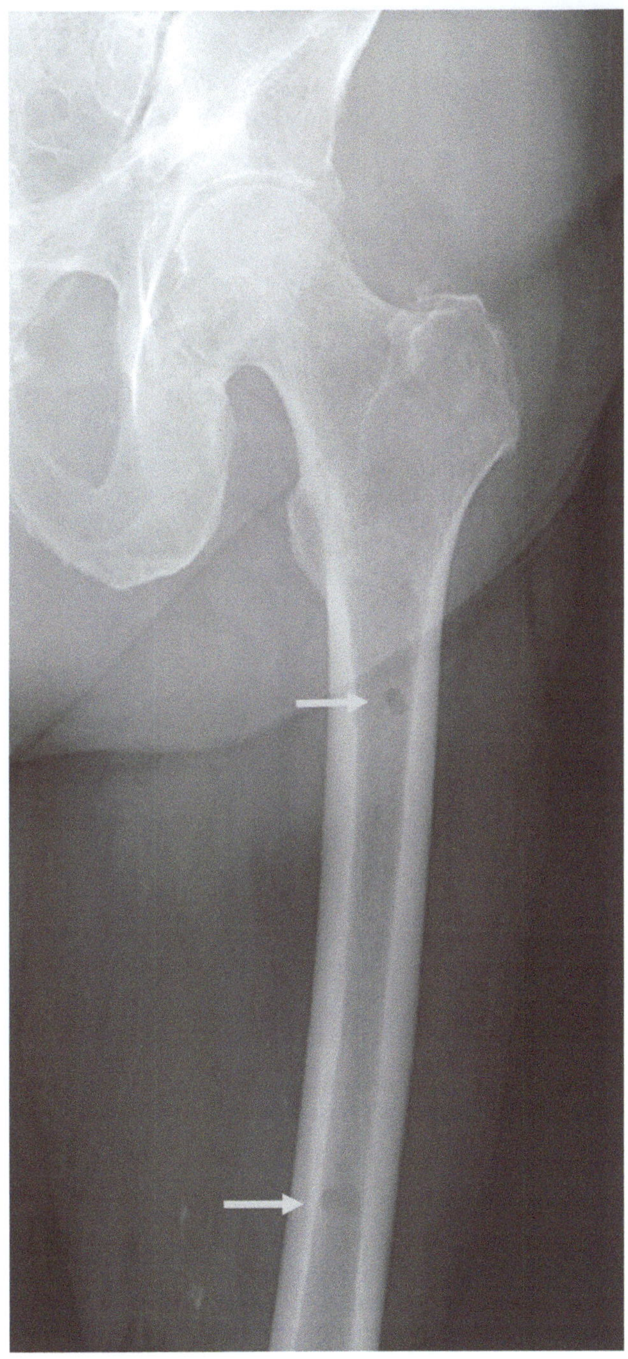

FIGURE 6.5 Lytic foci (*arrows*) without surrounding sclerosis in this femur are typical of multiple myeloma lesions.

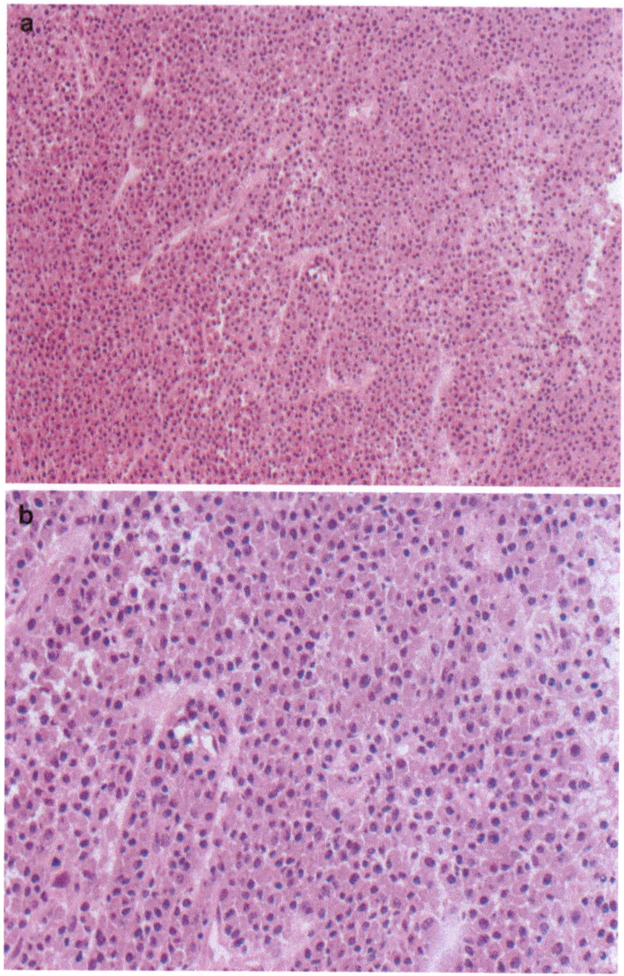

FIGURE 6.6 Low (**a**), intermediate (**b**), and high (**c**) power magnification of a case of multiple myeloma in which the sheets of neoplastic plasma cells can be easily identified.

various stages of development (Fig. 6.6). The main differential diagnosis is often other hematolymphoid neoplasms; however, myeloma cells are occasionally quite anaplastic and, as such, can easily mimic high-grade carcinoma and high-grade sarcoma.

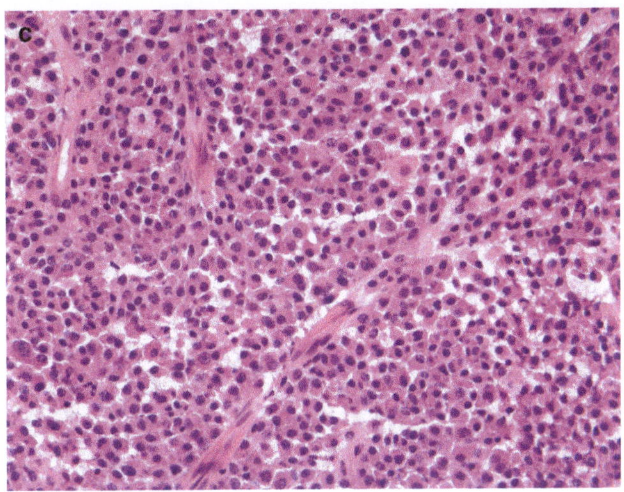

FIGURE 6.6   (continued)

Given that plasma cells and precursors may be easier to discern on intraoperative touch preparations stained by Romanowsky-type stains (e.g., Diff-Quick), it is strongly recommended that such an evaluation be always performed when plasmacytoma/myeloma and its mimickers are in the differential diagnosis.

OSTEOMYELITIS

Although this is a relatively common bone affliction, osteomyelitis is infrequently submitted for intraoperative evaluation, as the diagnosis is often made preoperatively based on the clinical and radiological findings. Early cases are associated with increased radionuclide uptake on bone scans; mixed sclerosis and radiolucency tend to appear later. Histologically, there is an acute inflammatory infiltrate composed predominantly of polymorphonuclear leukocytes with various degrees of marrow fibrosis; as cases become more chronic an associated plasma cell infiltrate is often also present (Fig. 6.7). Osteonecrosis, manifested as bone trabeculae with empty lacunae, as well as new bone formation is also frequently evident (Fig. 6.8), especially as these lesions age. Differential diagnostic considerations include the small round cell

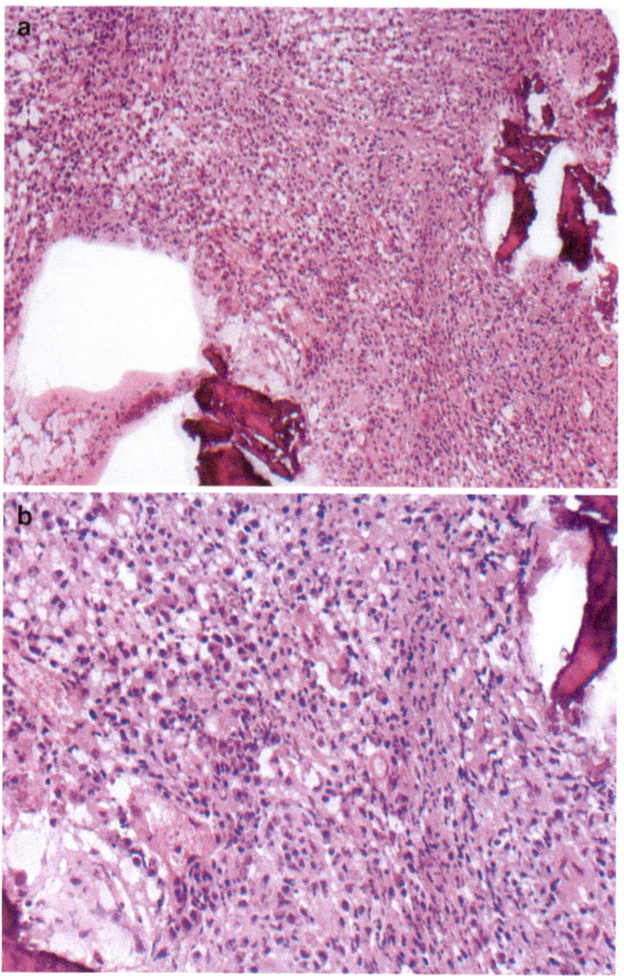

FIGURE 6.7 A case of osteomyelitis in which one observes a sheet of mixed inflammatory cells in between portions of mineralized bone (**a–c**).

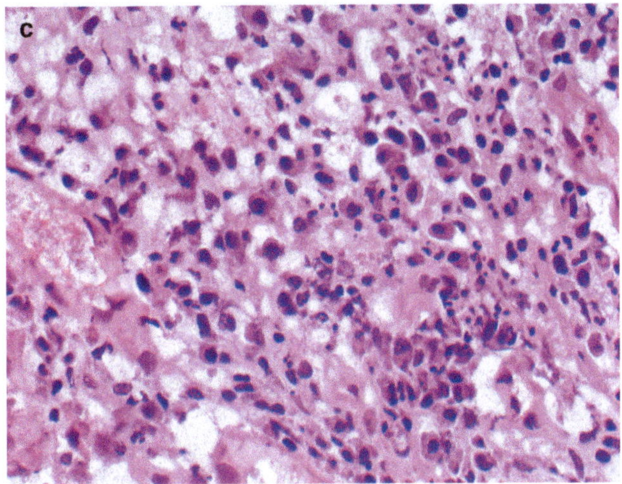

FIGURE 6.7   (continued)

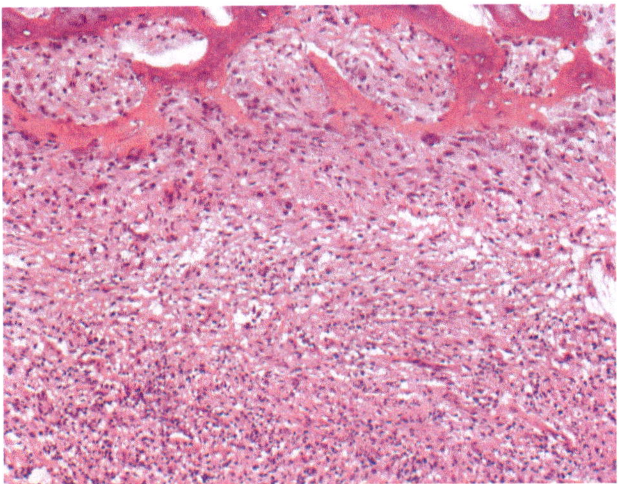

FIGURE 6.8   Another case of osteomyelitis in which there is new bone formation. This is evident as trabeculae of woven bone in the upper portion of the image.

tumors discussed above as well as LCH. Apart from the clinical and radiological findings and the fact that these conditions are unlikely to be associated with osteonecrosis, a monotonous population of cells would favor a round cell tumor, whereas intermixed eosinophils, histiocytes, and cells with characteristic morphology (see below) would favor LCH. Moreover, new bone formation would also be unusual in these conditions unless a fracture has occurred (see Chap. 2).

LANGERHANS CELL HISTIOCYTOSIS

This comprises a group of neoplastic Langerhans cell proliferations, all of which being capable of producing bone lesions. Such lesions can be unifocal (previously labeled solitary eosinophilic granuloma), multifocal (Hand–Schuller–Christian disease), or disseminated (Letterer–Siwe disease). The latter is thought by most to be a different entity – malignant histiocytosis). The craniofacial bones are most frequently affected, but LCH may also involve other bones such as the femur, pelvis, and ribs. Radiographically, lesions of LCH are radiolucent, often destructive and, in long bones, sometimes associated with exuberant periosteal new bone formation. Histologically, there is a mixed inflammatory infiltrate including neutrophils, eosinophils, lymphocytes, and histiocytes (with or without giant cells) in which Langerhans cells are identified (Fig. 6.9). These are cells with eosinophilic to clear cytoplasm containing oval, grooved, or multilobated nuclei (Fig. 6.10). Because of the histologic similarity to chronic osteomyelitis, lesions should be cultured, and the culture results should be known prior to formulating a final diagnosis.

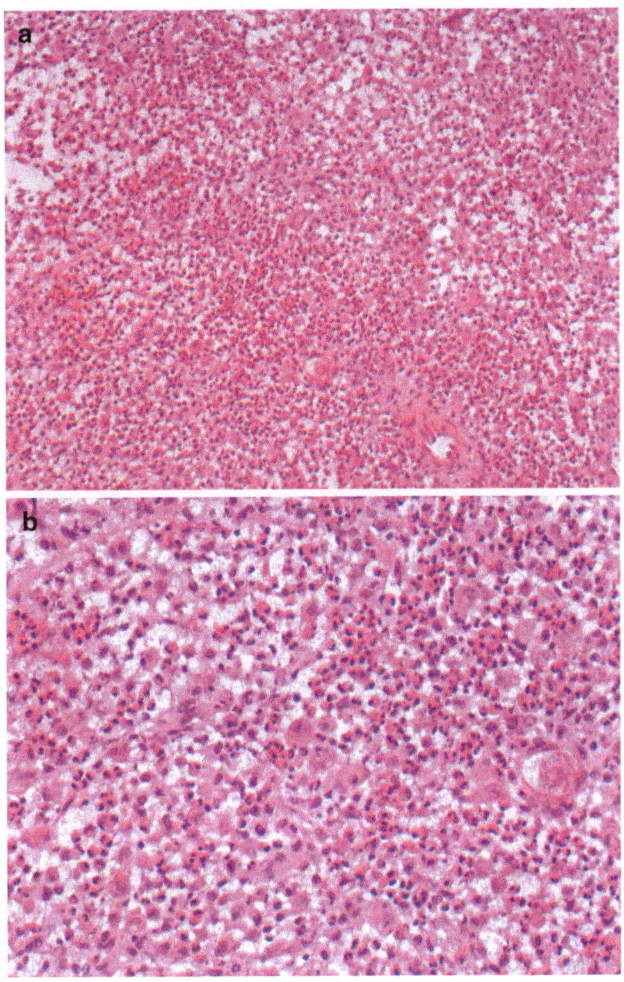

FIGURE 6.9 A case of Langerhans cell histiocytois characterized by abundant eosinophilic infiltration (**a**, **b**) among other component cells.

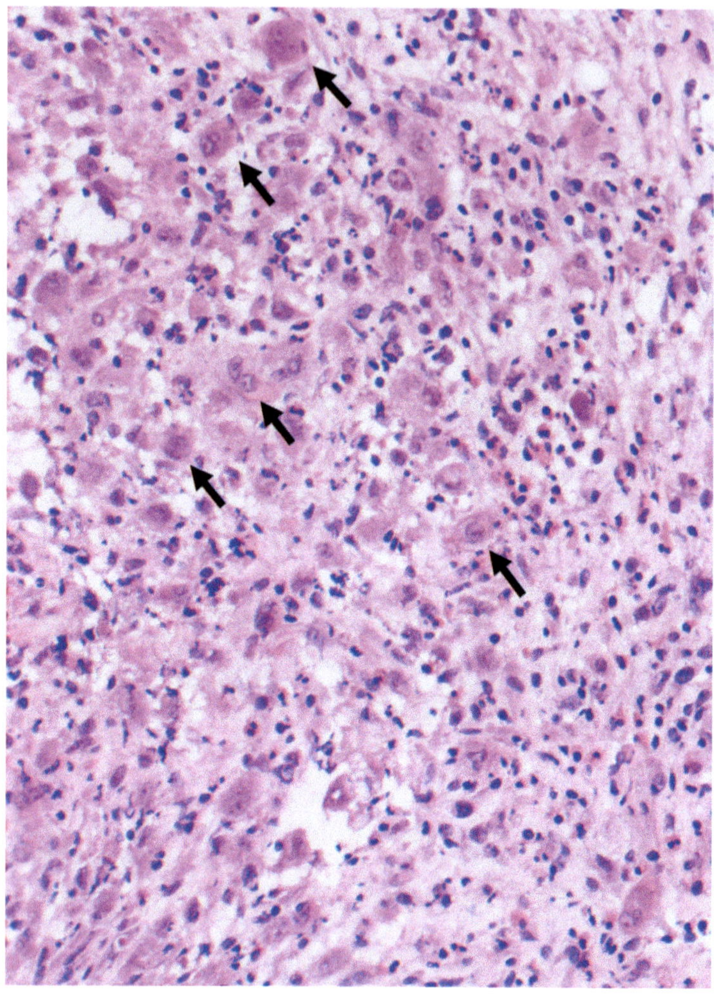

FIGURE 6.10 Another case of Langerhans cell histiocytois with less dense inflammatory infiltrate and fewer eosinophils. Notice the grooved and multinucleated Langerhans cells (*arrows*).

Chapter 7
Cystic and Vascular Lesions

INTRODUCTION

Since aneurysmal bone cyst has already been covered with other giant cell-containing lesions, the other cystic lesions that will be discussed in this chapter have been limited to simple bone cyst and intraosseus ganglion. Given the rarity of true vascular lesions of the bone only hemangioma, hemangioendothelioma, and angiosarcoma are referenced.

UNICAMERAL (SIMPLE) BONE CYST

Patients with this lesion usually present within the first two decades of life, most frequently with a pathological fracture, with the proximal humerus, femur, or tibia being the commonest sites of involvement. Radiologically, the lesion is circumscribed, radiolucent, and, unless there has been a fracture with displacement prior to healing, tends to be symmetric and without expansion of the bone or deformity. Unicameral bone cysts are usually lined by a thin fibrous membrane rarely covered by flattened cells of unknown type (Fig. 7.1). Such cells are often not visible on frozen section evaluation, but nonspecific findings including granulation tissue with chronic inflammation, cholesterol crystals, and hemosiderin deposition are usually evident (Fig. 7.1a, b). Because of this, the diagnosis (even on permanent sections) is one of exclusion and depends upon the presence of compatible radiological and operative findings, and the absence of histological features that might otherwise suggest an alternative diagnosis.

99

O. Hameed et al., *Frozen Section Library: Bone*, Frozen Section Library,
DOI 10.1007/978-1-4419-8376-3_7, © Springer Science+Business Media, LLC 2011

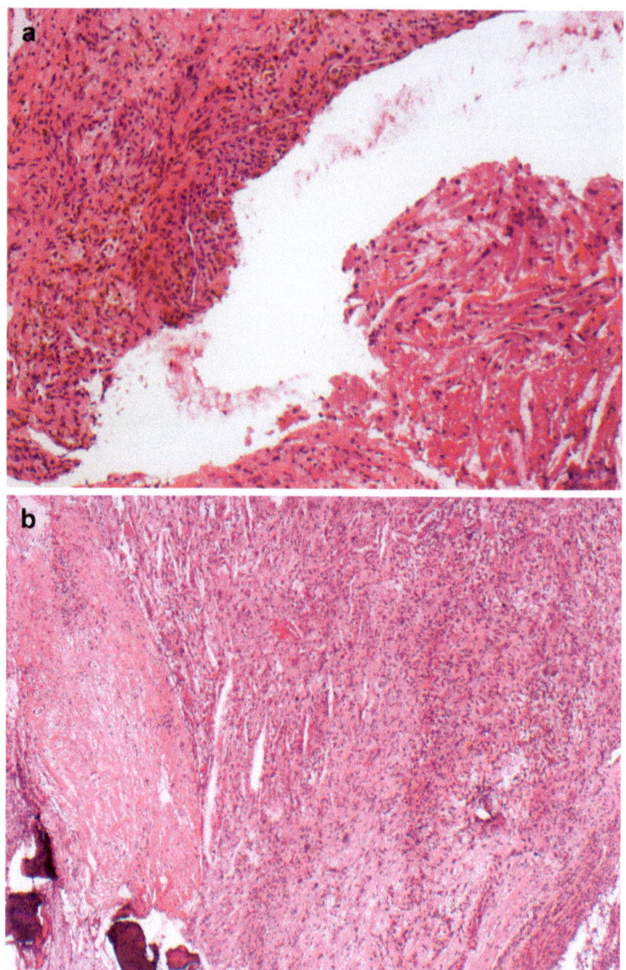

FIGURE 7.1 A unicameral (simple) bone cyst showing a cyst wall structure focally lined by flattened cells with underlying fibrosis and hemosiderin deposition (**a**). Cholesterol clefts are also evident, more so elsewhere in the lesion (**b**).

INTRAOSSEUS GANGLION CYST

This is an intramedullary, mucin-filled lesion that usually involves the epiphysis of select bones, most typically the tibia and femur and can arise at any age. Similar to its soft tissue counterpart, one may identify fibrous septae with myxoid matrix and mucin on frozen sectioning (Fig. 7.2).

HEMANGIOMA

Although incidental hemangiomas of bone are relatively common, clinically symptomatic tumors account for less than 1% of primary bone tumors. Such hemangiomas tend to present in late adulthood with the vertebral column being the most frequently involved site followed by the craniofacial skeleton and metaphyses of long bones. Hemangioma often appears on conventional radiographs as a vertically striate, "corduroy pattern" lesion in intact vertebrae, and as a radiolucent, often expansive lesion in long bones. Histologically, it is composed of capillary sized or cavernous vessels that permeate the marrow and are lined by bland endothelial cells (Fig. 7.3). It should be noted that this lesion is closely related to lymphangioma and it sometimes very difficult to distinguish between the two even on permanent sections without the use of immunohistochemistry.

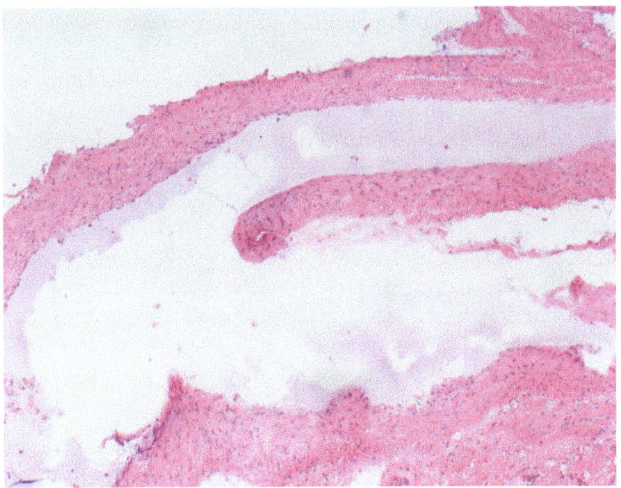

FIGURE 7.2 Intraosseous ganglion cyst showing bland fibrous septa and mucinous fluid.

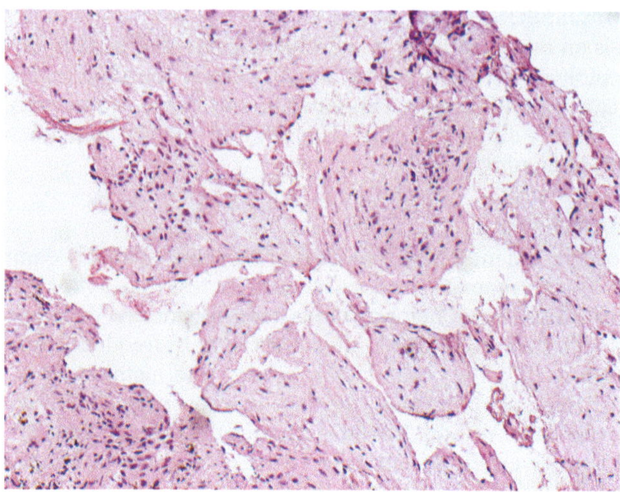

FIGURE 7.3   An example of an intraosseus hemangioma showing endothelial-lined vascular spaces.

ANGIOSARCOMA AND HEMANGIOENDOTHELIOMA

These two primary vascular neoplasms account for less than 1% of all bone tumors. Although they may present at any age group, the peak incidence is in young adulthood. They constitute a spectrum of lesions ranging from locally destructive, indolent tumors with a good response to surgery or local radiation to poorly differentiated malignant tumors with a high-metastatic rate. Most tumors are radiolucent with poor margination; however, a sclerotic rim is occasionally identified. While angiosarcomas are often solitary, hemangioendotheliomas tend to present as multifocal lesions in the same bone or in the same limb and, as such, may be mistaken for skeletal metastases. Histologically, angiosarcomas are usually characterized by the presence of irregularly anastomosing vascular channels lined by highly atypical endothelial cells, but, as do some hemangioendotheliomas, may only appear as aggregates or sheets of polyhedral or spindle cells without readily identified vascular spaces, especially on frozen sections (Fig. 7.4). The presence of cords,

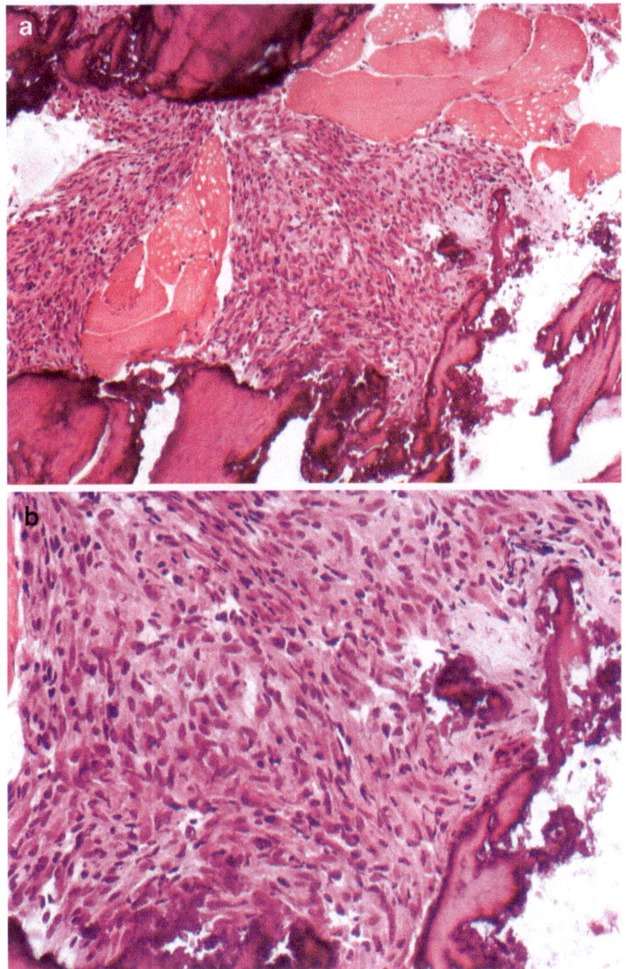

FIGURE 7.4   A case of spindle-cell hemangioendothelioma in which frozen sections (**a**, **b**) showed a cellular spindle-cell proliferation. The diagnosis was deferred. The vascular nature of the lesion became apparent on permanent sections (**c**, **d**).

nests, or sheets of plump vacuolated cells (± intracytoplasmic red blood cells), especially when the characteristic extracellular myxoid/hyalinized stroma is present, should suggest epithelioid hemangioendothelioma.

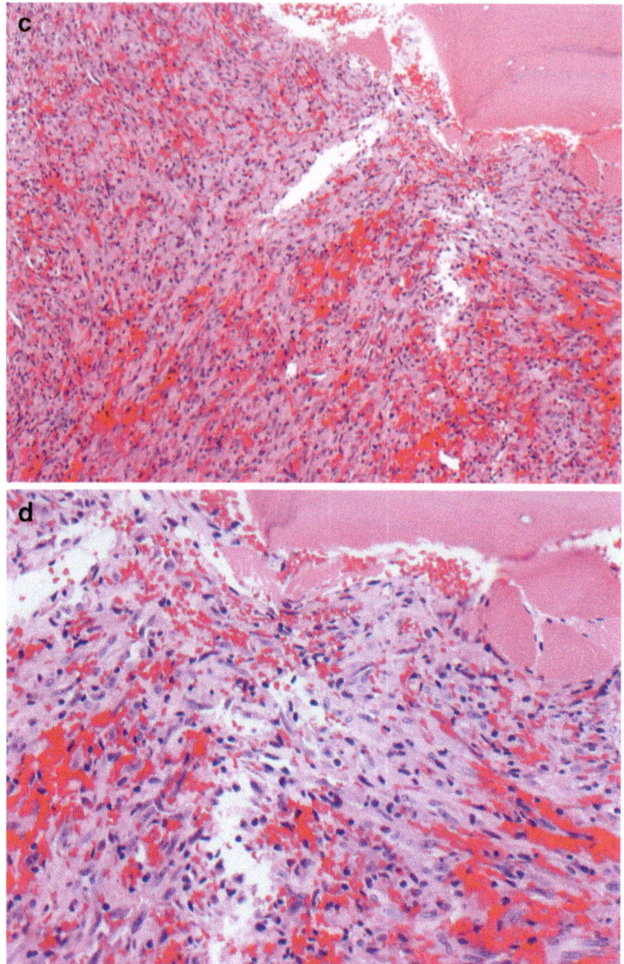

Figure 7.4 (continued)

Chapter 8
Epithelial Lesions

INTRODUCTION

INTRODUCTION

Although metastatic carcinoma represents the commonest epithelial lesion that can arise in bone, there are at least two primary bone neoplasms, namely adamantinoma and chordoma, that one should always consider these before making a diagnosis of metastatic carcinoma.

ADAMANTINOMA

This tumor comprises less than 1% of malignant bone tumors with the tibia being the most frequently involved site, followed by the fibula or both. There is a wide age distribution but the median age of patients is between 25 and 35 years. The lesion appears radiolucent and predominantly intracortical but may also involve the medullary cavity. Histologically, classic adamantinoma is composed of epithelial cells having a basaloid, tubular, or squamoid appearance; a predominantly spindle-cell pattern as well as mixtures of the above cell types can also be seen. A storiform fibroblastic proliferation that contains variable amounts of woven or lamellar bone may also be present. Rarely, the tumor is predominantly composed of the latter component, with only rare scattered epithelial cells. Thus, as discussed in Chap. 4, the findings can significantly overlap with those of osteofibrous dysplasia, with such cases described as having an "osteofibrous dysplasia-like pattern" or as "differentiated adamantinomas." As noted above, the main issue is not to misdiagnose this lesion as metastatic carcinoma and to keep this entity in mind when a tibial/fibular lesion with the appropriate morphology is being evaluated.

O. Hameed et al., *Frozen Section Library: Bone*, Frozen Section Library,
DOI 10.1007/978-1-4419-8376-3_8, © Springer Science+Business Media, LLC 2011

CHORDOMA

Although chordomas have traditionally been thought to be derived from notochordal remnants, they display epithelial differentiation, hence their inclusion in this chapter. Chordomas represent 4% of malignant bone tumors with most cases presenting after 30 years of age; the peak incidence is between 50 and 60 years. The "ends" of the spinal column in the axial skeleton, particularly the sacrum and the base of the skull, are usually affected. On imaging, they appear radiolucent with scattered calcifications; an associated soft tissue component is also frequently present. Histologically, chordomas are composed of lobules of tumor in which sheets, cords, or nests of vacuolated, eosinophilic to clear cells with abundant cytoplasm (physaliphorous cells) are seen embedded in myxoid matrix (Fig. 8.1). These appearances, along with the characteristic clinical and radiological findings, are usually sufficient to point toward the correct diagnosis during intraoperative evaluation. Because of the presence of areas that can mimic hyaline cartilage, however, the correct identification of so-called "chondroid" chordomas during frozen section evaluation (Fig. 8.2) is often more difficult. In fact, immunohistochemistry is frequently utilized in this situation to arrive at the correct diagnosis. Of note, the focal presence of a high-grade sarcomatous component should not necessarily point to an alternative diagnosis as dedifferentiated chordomas exist.

METASTATIC CARCINOMA

Metastatic carcinomas are the most common tumor affecting the skeleton. Moreover, the skeleton is the third most common site to be involved by metastatic tumor after the lungs and liver. Radiologically, metastatic deposits can be radiolucent, radiodense, or display a mixed sclerotic–lytic pattern. Given their high incidence, one should always consider metastatic carcinoma in the differential diagnosis of solitary or multiple bone lesions in patients over 40 years. Apart from the fact that metastatic carcinomas usually show evidence of epithelial differentiation, the histology usually resembles that of the primary carcinoma. Those of the breast (Fig. 8.3), lung (Figs. 8.4 and 8.5), prostate, kidney (Figs. 8.6 and 8.7), and thyroid gland (Fig. 8.8) comprise more than 80% of all bone metastases, but obviously many other

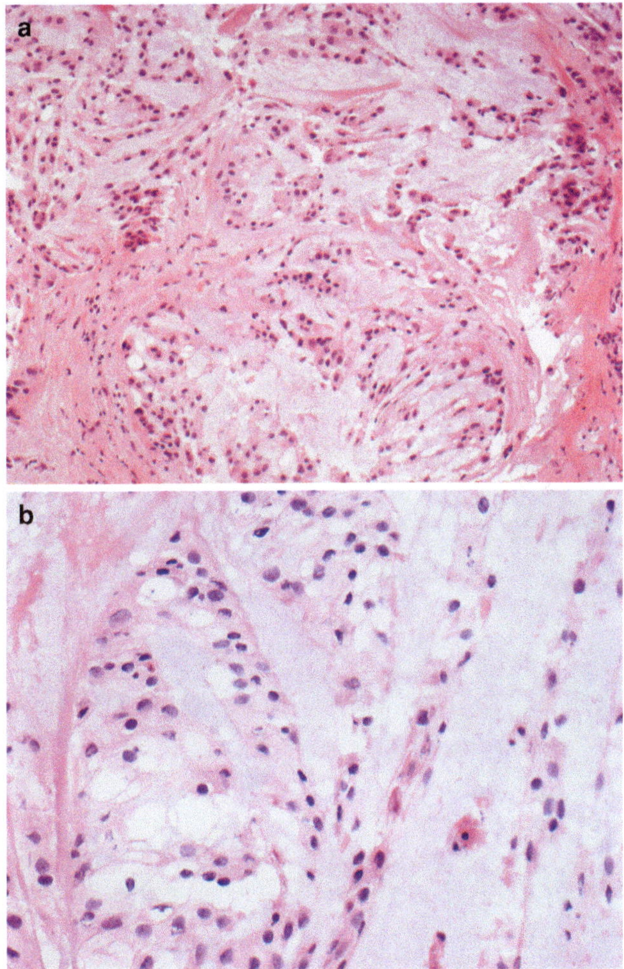

FIGURE 8.1   A frozen section of a chordoma (**a**, **b**) showing cords of tumor cells embedded in a myxoid matrix. Notice the characteristically abundant cytoplasm of the tumor cells (**b**).

malignant tumors (carcinomas or otherwise) can metastasize to the bone and be encountered intraoperatively. Although the histology is sometimes distinctive enough to suggest the primary origin even in the absence of a prior history (e.g., renal cell carcinoma; Fig. 8.6), in many cases the degree of frozen section artifacts

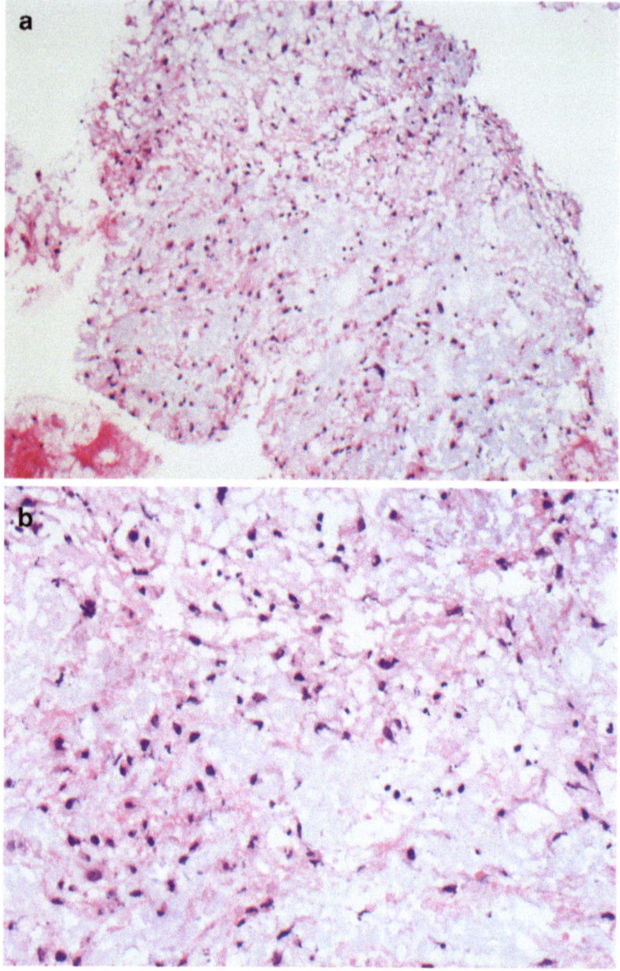

FIGURE 8.2 As depicted in this case, the appearances of chordoid chordoma on frozen sections (**a**, **b**) can significantly overlap with those of chondrosarcoma.

(Fig. 8.9) precludes making a more definitive diagnosis other than metastatic carcinoma. Because a prominent inflammatory, fibroblastic, osteoblastic, and/or vascular response may also obscure tumor cells, there should always be a high index of suspicion of

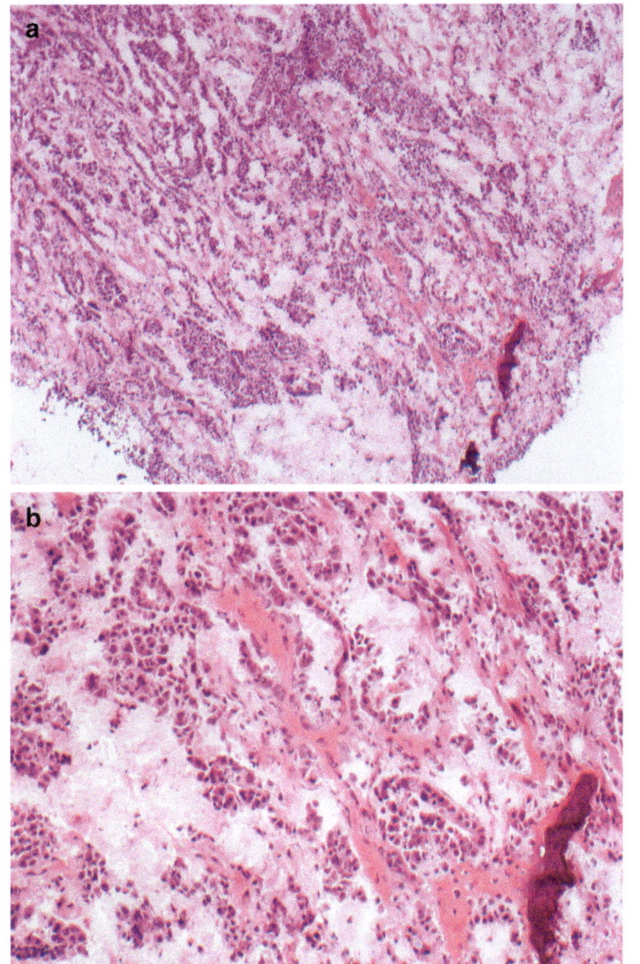

FIGURE 8.3 Low (**a**) and intermediate (**b**) power magnifications of a metastatic breast carcinoma within bone. Although the morphology here is certainly consistent with a breast primary, it is not sufficiently distinctive for such a definitive diagnosis in the absence of any prior history.

metastatic disease and, in the appropriate clinical and radiological setting, a careful search for occult neoplastic cells should always be undertaken, supplemented as necessary by immunohistochemical evaluation of paraffin-embedded material.

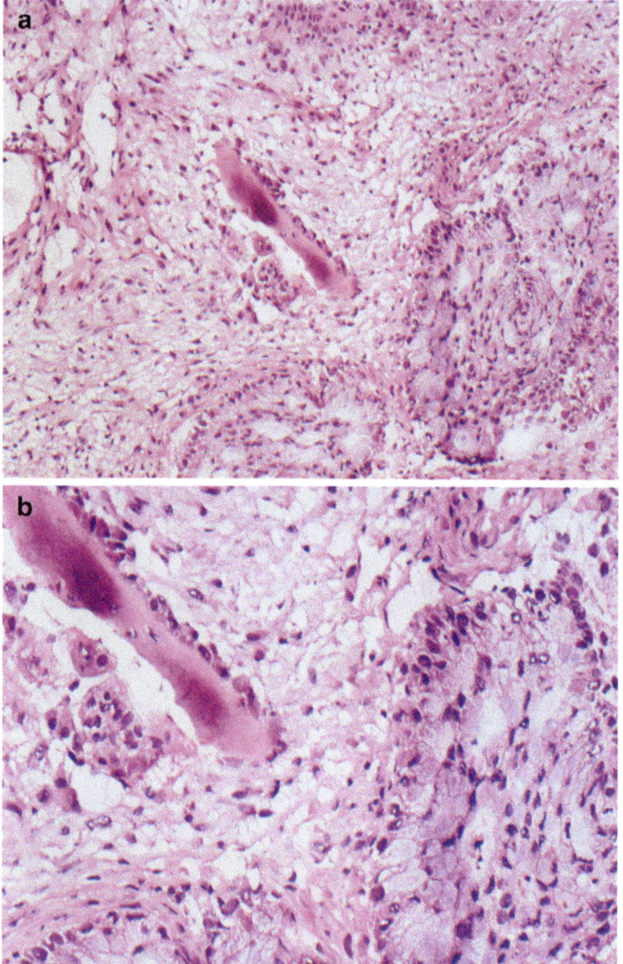

FIGURE 8.4 The morphology of this metastatic adenocarcinoma (**a**, **b**) also does not suggest a specific primary site. Nevertheless, the presence of intracellular mucin is compatible with the patient's history of a primary mucinous adenocarcinoma of the lung.

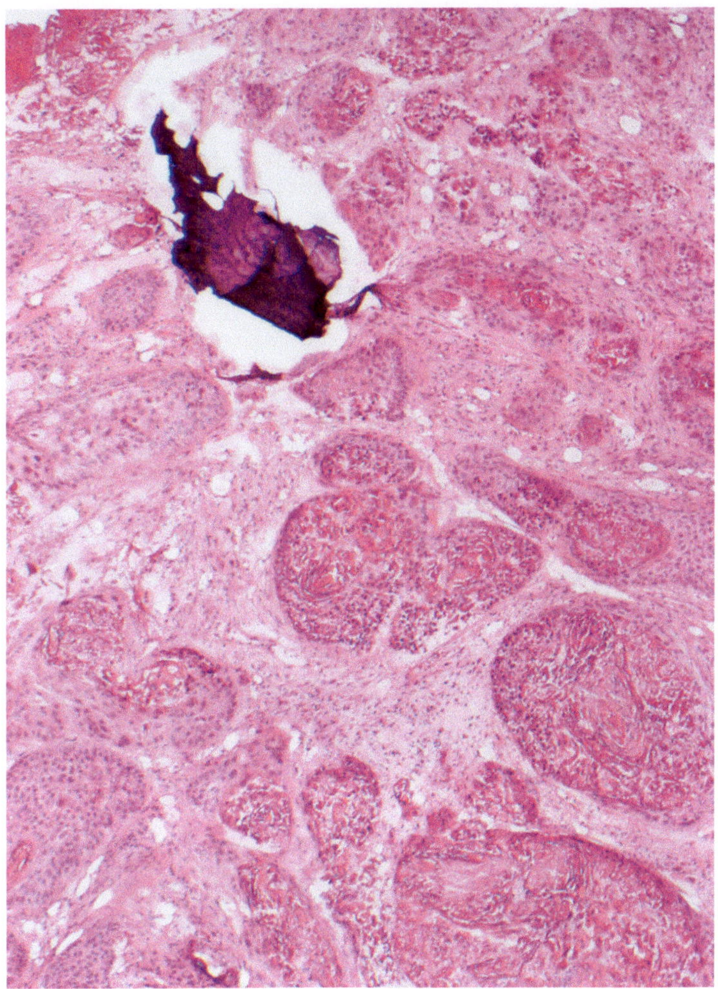

FIGURE 8.5 Another metastatic carcinoma of lung origin but here with squamous differentiation.

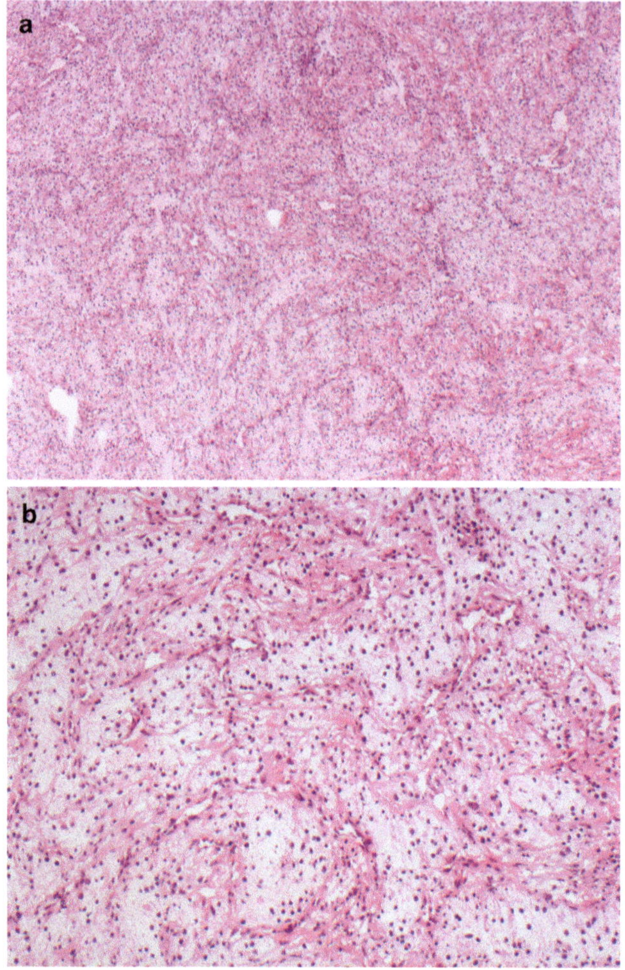

Figure 8.6 Although the low-power view (**a**) of this lesion may suggest an inflammatory process, the clear cell nature of its component cells and the sinusoidal vascular pattern, both of which become evident on higher magnification (**b**, **c**), should certainly suggest a diagnosis of metastatic clear cell renal carcinoma.

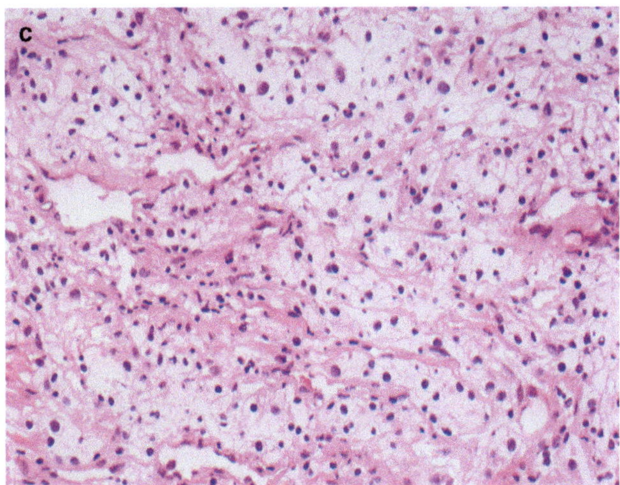

FIGURE 8.6 (continued)

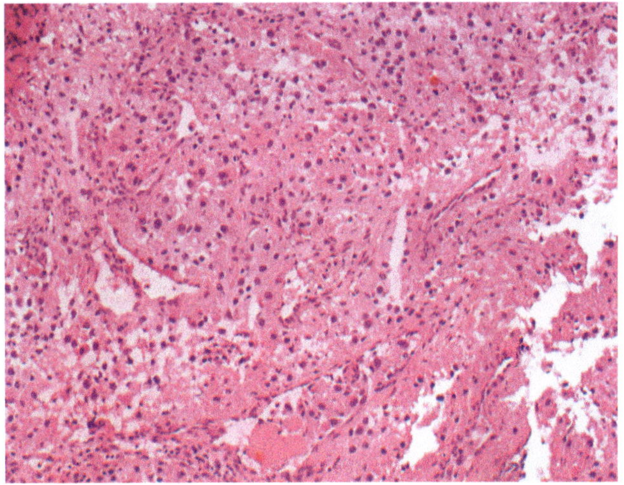

FIGURE 8.7 Another metastatic renal cell carcinoma characterized by dense eosinophilic cytoplasm rather than clear cells.

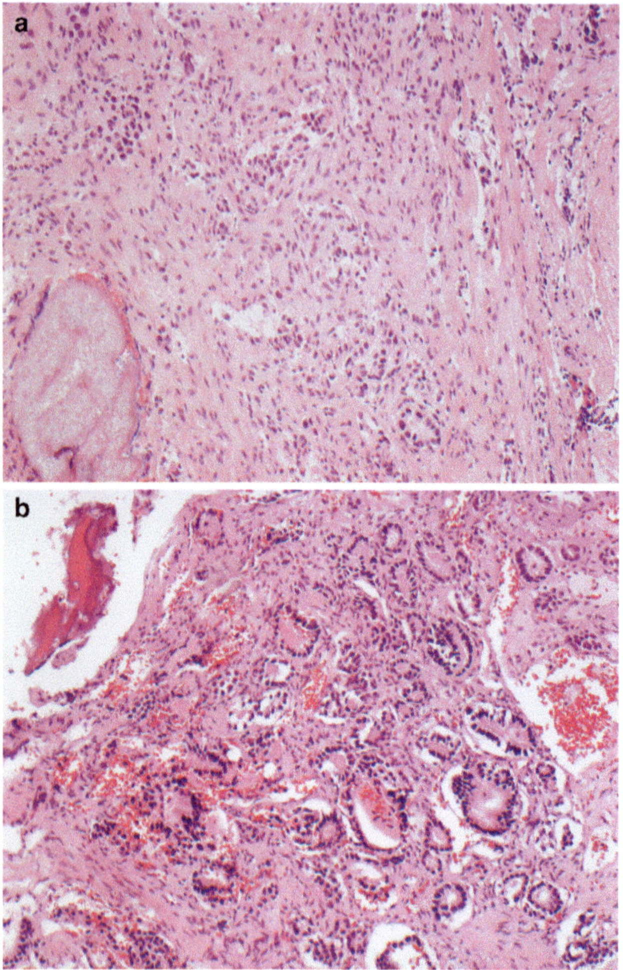

FIGURE 8.8 Metastatic thyroid carcinoma. The frozen section (**a**) displays scattered epithelial cells with some glandular formation; however, the presence of colloid within the glandular structures was only identified on permanent sections (**b**).

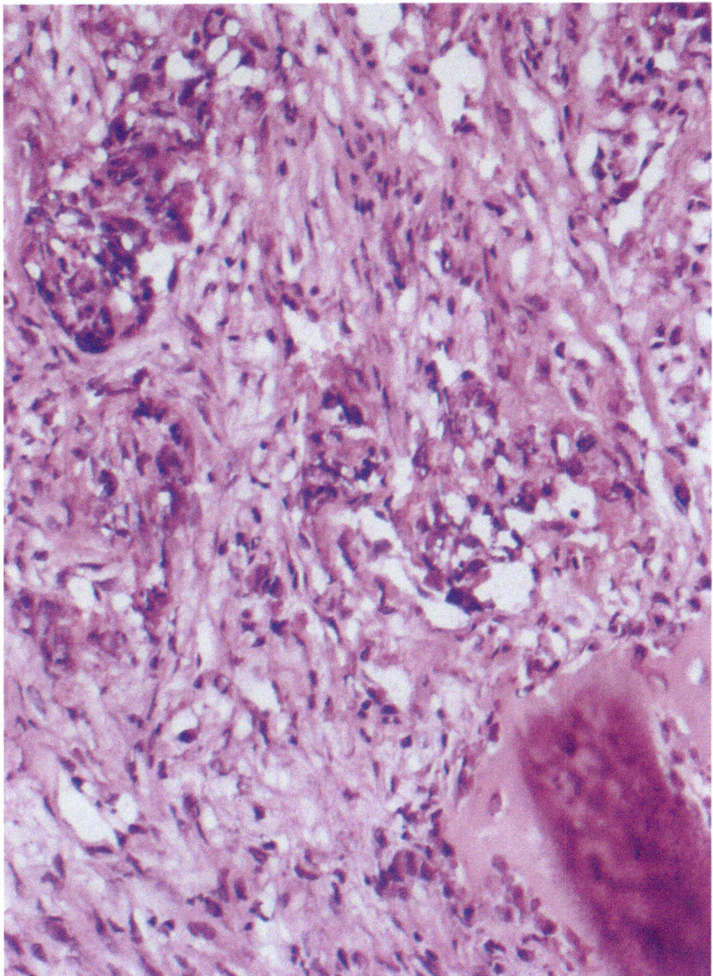

FIGURE 8.9 Metastatic colonic adenocarcinoma. Although suspicious for metastatic carcinoma, the degree of crushing/frozen section artifact present here would make this a tough diagnosis to make. In such cases, one should not hesitate to request for additional tissue and/or defer the diagnosis to permanent sections where immunohistochemistry or other special studies may help in identifying the correct site of origin.

Suggested Readings

General/Broad Topics

Abdul-Karim FW, Bauer TW, Kilpatrick SE, Raymond KA, Siegal GP, for the Association of Directors of Anatomic and Surgical Pathology. Recommendations for the reporting of bone tumors. Hum Pathol. 2004;35(10):1173–78.

Ackerman LV. Common errors made by pathologists in the diagnosis of bone tumors. Recent Results Cancer Res. 1976;(54):120–38.

Ayala AG, Raymond AK, Ro JY, Carrasco CH, Fanning CV, Murray JA. Needle biopsy of primary bone lesions. M.D. Anderson experience. Pathol Annu. 1989;24 Pt 1:219–51.

Bovée JV, Hogendoorn PC. Molecular pathology of sarcomas: concepts and clinical implications. Virchows Arch. 2010;456(2):193–99.

Brien EW, Mirra JM, Kerr R. Benign and malignant cartilage tumors of bone and joint: their anatomic and theoretical basis with an emphasis on radiology, pathology and clinical biology. I. The intramedullary cartilage tumors. Skeletal Radiol. 1997;26(6):325–53.

Bui MM, Smith P, Agresta SV, Cheong D, Letson GD. Practical issues of intraoperative frozen section diagnosis of bone and soft tissue lesions. Cancer Control. 2008;15(1):7–12.

Dahlin DC. Seventy-five years' experience with frozen sections at the Mayo Clinic. Mayo Clin Proc. 1980;55(11):721–23.

Deyrup AT, Montag AG. Epithelioid and epithelial neoplasms of bone. Arch Pathol Lab Med. 2007;131(2):205–16.

Dorfman HD, Czerniak B. Bone cancers. Cancer. 1995;75 (1 Suppl):203–10.

Horvai A, Unni KK. Premalignant conditions of bone. J Orthop Sci. 2006;11(4):412–23.

Huvos AG. Surgical pathology of bone sarcomas. World J Surg. 1988;12(3):284–98.

O. Hameed et al., *Frozen Section Library: Bone*, Frozen Section Library,
DOI 10.1007/978-1-4419-8376-3, © Springer Science+Business Media, LLC 2011

Johnson LC, Vinh TN, Sweet DE. Bone tumor dynamics: an orthopedic pathology perspective. Semin Musculoskelet Radiol. 2000;4(1):1–15.

Khuu H, Moore D, Young S, Jaffe KA, Siegal GP. Examination of tumor and tumor-like conditions of bone. Ann Diagn Pathol. 1999;3(6):364–69.

Li S, Siegal GP. Small cell tumors of bone. Adv Anat Pathol. 2010;17(1):1–11.

Miller TT. Bone tumors and tumorlike conditions: analysis with conventional radiography. Radiology. 2008;246(3):662–74.

Romeo S, Hogendoorn PC, Dei Tos AP. Benign cartilaginous tumors of bone: from morphology to somatic and germ-line genetics. Adv Anat Pathol. 2009;16(5):307–15.

Rubin BP, Antonescu CR, Gannon FH, Hunt JL, Inwards CY, Klein MJ, et al. Members of the Cancer Committee. College of American Pathologists. Protocol for the examination of specimens from patients with tumors of bone. Arch Pathol Lab Med. 2010;134(4):e1–7.

Schiller AL. Diagnosis of borderline cartilage lesions of bone. Semin Diagn Pathol. 1985;2(1):42–62.

Shah MS, Garg V, Kapoor SK, Dhaon BK, Gondal R. Fine-needle aspiration cytology, frozen section, and open biopsy: relative significance in diagnosis of musculoskeletal tumors. J Surg Orthop Adv. 2003;12(4):203–7.

Stacy GS, Mahal RS, Peabody TD. Staging of bone tumors: a review with illustrative examples. AJR Am J Roentgenol. 2006;186(4):967–76.

Unni KK. Cartilaginous lesions of bone. J Orthop Sci. 2001;6(5):457–72.

Unni KK, Dahlin DC. Grading of bone tumors. Semin Diagn Pathol. 1984;1(3):165–72.

Weatherby RP, Unni KK. Practical aspects of handling orthopedic specimens in the surgical pathology laboratory. Pathol Annu. 1982;17(Pt 2):1–31.

Aneurysmal Bone Cyst [ABC]

Campanacci M, Cervellati C, Donati U, Bertoni F. Aneurysmal bone cyst (a study of 127 cases, 72 with longterm follow up). Ital J Orthop Traumatol. 1976;2(3):341–53.

Cottalorda J, Bourelle S. Modern concepts of primary aneurysmal bone cyst. Arch Orthop Trauma Surg. 2007;127(2):105–14.

Martinez V, Sissons HA. Aneurysmal bone cyst. A review of 123 cases including primary lesions and those secondary to other bone pathology. Cancer. 1988;61(11):2291–304.

Oliveira AM, Perez-Atayde AR, Inwards CY, Medeiros F, Derr V, Hsi BL, et al. USP6 and CDH11 oncogenes identify the neoplastic cell in primary aneurysmal bone cysts and are absent in so-called secondary aneurysmal bone cysts. Am J Pathol. 2004;165(5):1773–80.

Vergel De Dios AM, Bond JR, Shives TC, McLeod RA, Unni KK. Aneurysmal bone cyst A clinicopathologic study of 238 cases. Cancer. 1992;69(12):2921–31.

Benign Fibrous Histiocytoma of Bone

Bertoni F, Calderoni P, Bacchini P, Sudanese A, Baldini N, Present D, et al. Benign fibrous histiocytoma of bone. J Bone Joint Surg Am. 1986;68(8):1225–30.

Clarke BE, Xipell JM, Thomas DP. Benign fibrous histiocytoma of bone. Am J Surg Pathol. 1985;9(11):806–15.

Grohs JG, Nicolakis M, Kainberger F, Lang S, Kotz R. Benign fibrous histiocytoma of bone: a report of ten cases and review of literature. Wien Klin Wochenschr. 2002;114(1–2):56–63.

Hamada T, Ito H, Araki Y, Fujii K, Inoue M, Ishida O. Benign fibrous histiocytoma of the femur: review of three cases. Skeletal Radiol. 1996;25(1):25–9.

Matsuno T. Benign fibrous histiocytoma involving the ends of long bone. Skeletal Radiol. 1990;19(8):561–66.

Roessner A, Immenkamp M, Weidner A, Hobik HP, Grundmann E. Benign fibrous histiocytoma of bone. Light- and electron-microscopic observations. J Cancer Res Clin Oncol. 1981;101(2):191–202.

Bizarre Parosteal Osteochondromatous Proliferations

Abramovici L, Steiner GC. Bizarre parosteal osteochondromatous proliferation (Nora's lesion): a retrospective study of 12 cases, 2 arising in long bones. Hum Pathol. 2002;33(12):1205–10.

Campanacci DA, Guarracino R, Franchi A, Capanna R. Bizarre parosteal osteochondromatous proliferation (Nora's lesion). Description of six cases and a review of the literature. Chir Organi Mov. 1999;84(1):65–71.

deLange EE, Pope Jr TL, Fechner RE, Keats TE. Bizarre parosteal osteochondromatous proliferation vs. benign florid reactive periostitis. AJR Am J Roentgenol. 1987;148(3):650.

Meneses MF, Unni KK, Swee RG. Bizarre parosteal osteochondromatous proliferation of bone (Nora's lesion). Am J Surg Pathol. 1993;17(7):691–97.

Nora FE, Dahlin DC, Beabout JW. Bizarre parosteal osteochondromatous proliferations of the hands and feet. Am J Surg Pathol. 1983;7(3):245–50.

Brown Tumor of Bone [Hyperparathyroidism]

Diamanti-Kandarakis E, Livadas S, Tseleni-Balafouta S, Lyberopoulos K, Tantalaki E, Palioura H, et al. Brown tumor of the fibula: unusual presentation of an uncommon manifestation. Report of a case and review of the literature. Endocrine. 2007;32(3):345–49.

Galvin AH. Osteitis fibrosa cystica occurring in a flat bone: report of a case. Cal State J Med. 1923;21(6):244–45.

Pavlovic S, Valyi-Nagy T, Profirovic J, David O. Fine-needle aspiration of brown tumor of bone: cytologic features with radiologic and histologic correlation. Diagn Cytopathol. 2009;37(2):136–39.

Chondroblastoma

Bertoni F, Unni KK, Beabout JW, Harner SG, Dahlin DC. Chondroblastoma of the skull and facial bones. Am J Clin Pathol. 1987;88(1):1–9.

Dahlin DC, Ivins JC. Benign chondroblastoma. A study of 125 cases. Cancer. 1972;30(2):401–13.

Forest M, De Pinieux G. Chondroblastoma and its differential diagnosis. Ann Pathol. 2001;21(6):468–78.

Huvos AG, Marcove RC. Chondroblastoma of bone. A critical review. Clin Orthop Relat Res. 1973;(95):300–12.

Marcove RC, Alpert M. A pathologic study of benign osteoblastoma. Clin Orthop Relat Res. 1963;30:175–81.

Springfield DS, Capanna R, Gherlinzoni F, Picci P, Campanacci M. Chondroblastoma. A review of seventy cases. J Bone Joint Surg Am. 1985;67(5):748–55.

[En]Chondroma

Bonnevialle P, Mansat M, Durroux R, Devallet P, Rongières M. Chondromas of the hand. A report of thirty-five cases. Ann Chir Main. 1988;7(1):32–44.

Jones KB, Buckwalter JA, Frassica FJ, McCarthy EF. Intracortical chondroma: a report of two cases. Skeletal Radiol. 2006;35(5):298–301.

Lewis MM, Kenan S, Yabut SM, Norman A, Steiner G. Periosteal chondroma. A report of ten cases and review of the literature. Clin Orthop Relat Res. 1990;(256):185–92.

Marcozzi G, Messinetti S. Maffucci's syndrome in its clinical, radiological, anatomical, pathological and pathogenetic aspects; dyschondroplasia with multiple angiomas. Ann Ital Chir. 1956;33(6):504–33.

McFarland Jr GB, Morden ML. Benign cartilaginous lesions. Orthop Clin North Am. 1977;8(4):737–49.

Mirra JM, Gold R, Downs J, Eckardt JJ. A new histologic approach to the differentiation of enchondroma and chondrosarcoma of the bones. A clinicopathologic analysis of 51 cases. Clin Orthop Relat Res. 1985;(201):214–37.

Umansky AL. Dyschondroplasia with hemangiomata (Maffucci's syndrome); report of an early case with mild osseous manifestations. Bull Hosp Joint Dis. 1946;7(1):59–68.

Chondromyxoid Fibroma

Baker AC, Rezeanu L, O'Laughlin S, Unni K, Klein MJ, Siegal GP. Juxtacortical chondromyxoid fibroma of bone: a unique variant: a case study of 20 patients. Am J Surg Pathol. 2007;31(11):1662–68.

Jaffe HL, Lichtenstein L. Chondromyxoid fibroma of bone; a distinctive benign tumor likely to be mistaken especially for chondrosarcoma. Arch Pathol. 1948;45(4):541–51.

Nielsen GP, Keel SB, Dickersin GR, Selig MK, Bhan AK, Rosenberg AE. Chondromyxoid fibroma: a tumor showing myofibroblastic, myochondroblastic, and chondrocytic differentiation. Mod Pathol. 1999; 12(5):514–17.

Rahimi A, Beabout JW, Ivins JC, Dahlin DC. Chondromyxoid fibroma: a clinicopathologic study of 76 cases. Cancer. 1972;30(3):726–36.

Wu CT, Inwards CY, O'Laughlin S, Rock MG, Beabout JW, Unni KK. Chondromyxoid fibroma of bone: a clinicopathologic review of 278 cases. Hum Pathol. 1998;29(5):438–46.

Yamaguchi T, Dorfman HD. Radiographic and histologic patterns of calcification in chondromyxoid fibroma. Skeletal Radiol. 1998;27(10):559–64.

Zillmer DA, Dorfman HD. Chondromyxoid fibroma of bone: thirty-six cases with clinicopathologic correlation. Hum Pathol. 1989;20(10):952–64.

Chondrosarcoma

Bjornsson J, Unni KK, Dahlin DC, Beabout JW, Sim FH. Clear cell chondrosarcoma of bone. Observations in 47 cases. Am J Surg Pathol. 1984; 8(3):223–30.

Chow WA. Update on chondrosarcomas. Curr Opin Oncol. 2007;19(4): 371–76.

Evans HL, Ayala AG, Romsdahl MM. Prognostic factors in chondrosarcoma of bone: a clinicopathologic analysis with emphasis on histologic grading. Cancer. 1977;40(2):818–31.

Frassica FJ, Unni KK, Beabout JW, Sim FH. Dedifferentiated chondrosarcoma. A report of the clinicopathological features and treatment of seventy-eight cases. J Bone Joint Surg Am. 1986;68(8):1197–205.

Gitelis S, Bertoni F, Picci P, Campanacci M. Chondrosarcoma of bone. The experience at the Istituto Ortopedico Rizzoli. J Bone Joint Surg Am. 1981;63(8):1248–57.

Lichtenstein L, Jaffe HL. Chondrosarcoma of bone. Am J Pathol. 1943;19(4):553–89.

Pritchard DJ, Lunke RJ, Taylor WF, Dahlin DC, Medley BE. Chondrosarcoma: a clinicopathologic and statistical analysis. Cancer. 1980;45(1):149–57.

Skeletal Lesions Interobserver Correlation among Expert Diagnosticians (SLICED) Study Group. Reliability of histopathologic and radiologic grading of cartilaginous neoplasms in long bones. J Bone Joint Surg Am. 2007;89(10):2113–23.

Unni KK, Dahlin DC, Beabout JW, Sim FH. Chondrosarcoma: clear-cell variant. A report of sixteen cases. J Bone Joint Surg Am. 1976a;58(5):676–83.

Chordoma

Chambers PW, Schwinn CP. Chordoma. A clinicopathologic study of metastasis. Am J Clin Pathol. 1979;72(5):765–76.

Chugh R, Tawbi H, Lucas DR, Biermann JS, Schuetze SM, Baker LH. Chordoma: the nonsarcoma primary bone tumor. Oncologist. 2007; 12(11):1344–50.

Dahlin DC, Unni KK. Chordoma. Arch Pathol Lab Med. 1994; 118(6):596–97.

Pamir MN, Ozduman K. Tumor-biology and current treatment of skull-base chordomas. Adv Tech Stand Neurosurg. 2008;33:35–129.

Riopel C, Michot C. Chordomas. Ann Pathol. 2007;27(1):6–15.

Rosenberg AE, Bhan AK, Lee JM. Chondroid chordoma. Am J Clin Pathol. 1995;104(4):484.

Sundaresan N, Galicich JH, Chu FC, Huvos AG. Spinal chordomas. J Neurosurg. 1979;50(3):312–19.

Ewing's Sarcoma/PNET

Askin FB, Rosai J, Sibley RK, Dehner LP, McAlister WH. Malignant small cell tumor of the thoracopulmonary region in childhood: a distinctive clinicopathologic entity of uncertain histogenesis. Cancer. 1979;43(6):2438–51.

Bacci G, Longhi A, Ferrari S, Mercuri M, Versari M, Bertoni F. Prognostic factors in non-metastatic Ewing's sarcoma tumor of bone: an analysis of 579 patients treated at a single institution with adjuvant or neoadjuvant chemotherapy between 1972 and 1998. Acta Oncol. 2006;45(4):469–75.

Iwamoto Y. Diagnosis and treatment of Ewing's sarcoma. Jpn J Clin Oncol. 2007;37(2):79–89.

Kissane JM, Askin FB, Foulkes M, Stratton LB, Shirley SF. Ewing's sarcoma of bone: clinicopathologic aspects of 303 cases from the Intergroup Ewing's Sarcoma Study. Hum Pathol. 1983;14(9):773–79.

Lichtenstein L, Jaffe HL. Ewing's sarcoma of bone. Am J Pathol. 1947;23(1):43–77.

Llombart-Bosch A, Machado I, Navarro S, Bertoni F, Bacchini P, Alberghini M, et al. Histological heterogeneity of Ewing's sarcoma/PNET: an immunohistochemical analysis of 415 genetically confirmed cases with clinical support. Virchows Arch. 2009;455(5):397–411.

Maheshwari AV, Cheng EY. Ewing sarcoma family of tumors. J Am Acad Orthop Surg. 2010;18(2):94–107.

Maygarden SJ, Askin FB, Siegal GP, Gilula LA, Schoppe J, Foulkes M, et al. Ewing sarcoma of bone in infants and toddlers. A clinicopathologic report from the Intergroup Ewing's Study. Cancer. 1993;71(6):2109–18.

Terrier P, Llombart-Bosch A, Contesso G. Small round blue cell tumors in bone: prognostic factors correlated to Ewing's sarcoma and neuroectodermal tumors. Semin Diagn Pathol. 1996;13(3):250–57.

Ushigome S, Shimoda T, Nikaido T, Nakamori K, Miyazawa Y, Shishikura A, et al. Primitive neuroectodermal tumors of bone and soft tissue. With reference to histologic differentiation in primary or metastatic foci. Acta Pathol Jpn. 1992;42(7):483–93.

Wilkins RM, Pritchard DJ, Burgert Jr EO, Unni KK. Ewing's sarcoma of bone. Experience with 140 patients. Cancer. 1986;58(11):2551–55.

Fibrosarcoma

Bertoni F, Capanna R, Calderoni P, Patrizia B, Campanacci M. Primary central (medullary) fibrosarcoma of bone. Semin Diagn Pathol. 1984;1(3):185–98.

Dahlin DC, Ivins JC. Fibrosarcoma of bone. A study of 114 cases. Cancer. 1969;23(1):35–41.

Huvos AG, Higinbotham NL. Primary fibrosarcoma of bone. A clinicopathologic study of 130 patients. Cancer. 1975;35(3):837–47.

Papagelopoulos PJ, Galanis EC, Trantafyllidis P, Boscainos PJ, Sim FH, Unni KK. Clinicopathologic features, diagnosis, and treatment of fibrosarcoma of bone. Am J Orthop. 2002;31(5):253–57.

Fibrous Dysplasia

Chapurlat RD, Orcel P. Fibrous dysplasia of bone and McCune-Albright syndrome. Best Pract Res Clin Rheumatol. 2008;22(1):55–69.

Jaffe HL. Fibrous dysplasia of bone. Bull NY Acad Med. 1946;22(11):588–604.

Jhala DN, Eltoum I, Carroll AJ, Lopez-Ben R, Lopez-Terrada D, Rao PH, et al. Osteosarcoma in a patient with McCune-Albright syndrome and Mazabraud's syndrome: a case report emphasizing the cytological and cytogenetic findings. Hum Pathol. 2003;34(12):1354–57.

Kyriakos M, McDonald DJ, Sundaram M. Fibrous dysplasia with cartilaginous differentiation ("fibrocartilaginous dysplasia"): a review, with an illustrative case followed for 18 years. Skeletal Radiol. 2004;33(1):51–62.

Pollandt K, Engels C, Kaiser E, Werner M, Delling G. Gs alpha gene mutations in monostotic fibrous dysplasia of bone and fibrous dysplasia-like low-grade central osteosarcoma. Virchows Arch. 2001;439(2):170–75.

Riminucci M, Robey PG, Bianco P. The pathology of fibrous dysplasia and the McCune-Albright syndrome. Pediatr Endocrinol Rev. 2007;4 Suppl 4:401–11.

Giant Cell Reparative Granuloma/Solid Variant ABC

Auclair PL, Cuenin P, Kratochvil FJ, Slater LJ, Ellis GL. A clinical and histomorpho logic comparison of the central giant cell granuloma and the giant cell tumor. Oral Surg Oral Med Oral Pathol. 1988;66(2):197–208.

Ilaslan H, Sundaram M, Unni KK. Solid variant of aneurysmal bone cysts in long tubular bones: giant cell reparative granuloma. AJR Am J Roentgenol. 2003;180(6):1681–87.

Ratner V, Dorfman HD. Giant-cell reparative granuloma of the hand and foot bones. Clin Orthop Relat Res. 1990;260:251–58.

Sanerkin NG, Mott MG, Roylance J. An unusual intraosseous lesion with fibroblastic, osteoclastic, osteoblastic, aneurysmal and fibromyxoid elements. "Solid" variant of aneurysmal bone cyst. Cancer. 1983;51(12):2278–86.

Wold LE, Dobyns JH, Swee RG, Dahlin DC. Giant cell reaction (giant cell reparative granuloma) of the small bones of the hands and feet. Am J Surg Pathol. 1986;10(7):491–96.

Yamaguchi T, Dorfman HD. Giant cell reparative granuloma: a comparative clinicopathologic study of lesions in gnathic and extragnathic sites. Int J Surg Pathol. 2001;9(3):189–200.

Giant Cell Tumor of Bone

Aegerter EE. Giant cell tumor of bone: a critical survey. Am J Pathol. 1947;23(2):283–97.

Campanacci M, Baldini N, Boriani S, Sudanese A. Giant-cell tumor of bone. J Bone Joint Surg Am. 1987;69(1):106–14.

Cummins CA, Scarborough MT, Enneking WF. Multicentric giant cell tumor of bone. Clin Orthop Relat Res. 1996;(322):245–52.

Dahlin DC. Caldwell lecture. Giant cell tumor of bone: highlights of 407 cases. AJR Am J Roentgenol. 1985;144(5):955–60.

Gupta R, Seethalakshmi V, Jambhekar NA, Prabhudesai S, Merchant N, Puri A, et al. Clinicopathologic profile of 470 giant cell tumors of bone from a cancer hospital in western India. Ann Diagn Pathol. 2008;12(4):239–48.

Lichtenstein L. Giant-cell tumor of bone; current status of problems in diagnosis and treatment. J Bone Joint Surg Am. 1951;33(A:1):143–50.

Wülling M, Engels C, Jesse N, Werner M, Delling G, Kaiser E. The nature of giant cell tumor of bone. J Cancer Res Clin Oncol. 2001;127(8):467–74.

Wold LE, Swee RG. Giant cell tumor of the small bones of the hands and feet. Semin Diagn Pathol. 1984;1(3):173–84.

Hemangioma/Hemangioendothelioma/Angiosarcoma of Bone

Dorfman HD, Steiner GC, Jaffe HL. Vascular tumors of bone. Hum Pathol. 1971;2(3):349–76.

Evans HL, Raymond AK, Ayala AG. Vascular tumors of bone: a study of 17 cases other than ordinary hemangioma, with an evaluation of the relationship of hemangio endothelioma of bone to epithelioid hemangioma, epithelioid hemangioendothel ioma, and high-grade angiosarcoma. Hum Pathol. 2003;34(7):680–89.

Kleer CG, Unni KK, McLeod RA. Epithelioid hemangioendothelioma of bone. Am J Surg Pathol. 1996;20(11):1301–11.

Nielsen GP, Srivastava A, Kattapuram S, Deshpande V, O'Connell JX, Mangham CD, et al. Epithelioid hemangioma of bone revisited: a study of 50 cases. Am J Surg Pathol. 2009;33(2):270–77.

O'Connell JX, Nielsen GP, Rosenberg AE. Epithelioid vascular tumors of bone: a review and proposal of a classification scheme. Adv Anat Pathol. 2001;8(2):74–82.

Tsuneyoshi M, Dorfman HD, Bauer TW. Epithelioid hemangioendothelioma of bone. A clinicopathologic, ultrastructural, and immunohistochemical study. Am J Surg Pathol. 1986;10(11):754–64.

Unni KK, Ivins JC, Beabout JW, Dahlin DC. Hemangioma, hemangiopericytoma, and hemangioendothelioma (angiosarcoma) of bone. Cancer. 1971;27(6):1403–14.

Wold LE, Unni KK, Beabout JW, Ivins JC, Bruckman JE, Dahlin DC. Hemangioendothelial sarcoma of bone. Am J Surg Pathol. 1982;6(1):59–70.

Langerhans' Cell Histiocytosis

Egeler RM, D'Angio GJ. Langerhans cell histiocytosis. J Pediatr. 1995;127(1):1–11.

Favara BE, McCarthy RC, Mierau GW. Histiocytosis X. Hum Pathol. 1983;14(8):663–76.

Jaffe R. Pathology of histiocytosis X. Perspect Pediatr Pathol. 1987;9:4–47.

Kilpatrick SE, Wenger DE, Gilchrist GS, Shives TC, Wollan PC, Unni KK. Langerhans' cell histiocytosis (histiocytosis X) of bone. A clinicopathologic analysis of 263 pediatric and adult cases. Cancer. 1995;76(12):2471–84.

Lichtenstein L. Histiocytosis X (eosinophilic granuloma of bone, Letterer-Siwe disease, and Schueller-Christian disease). Further observations of pathological and clinical importance. J Bone Joint Surg Am. 1964;46:76–90.

Lieberman PH, Jones CR, Steinman RM, Erlandson RA, Smith J, Gee T, et al. Langerhans cell (eosinophilic) granulomatosis. A clinicopathologic study encompassing 50 years. Am J Surg Pathol. 1996;20(5): 519–52.

Osband ME, Histiocytosis X. Langerhans' cell histiocytosis. Hematol Oncol Clin North Am. 1987;1(4):737–51.

Wester SM, Beabout JW, Unni KK, Dahlin DC. Langerhans' cell granulomatosis (histiocytosis X) of bone in adults. Am J Surg Pathol. 1982;6(5):413–26.

Leiomyosarcoma of Bone

Adelani MA, Schultenover SJ, Holt GE, Cates JM. Primary leiomyosarcoma of extragnathic bone: clinicopathologic features and reevaluation of prognosis. Arch Pathol Lab Med. 2009;133(9):1448–56.

Antonescu CR, Erlandson RA, Huvos AG. Primary leiomyosarcoma of bone: a clinicopathologic, immunohistochemical, and ultrastructural study of 33 patients and a literature review. Am J Surg Pathol. 1997;21(11):1281–94.

Berlin O, Angervall L, Kindblom LG, Berlin IC, Stener B. Primary leiomyosarcoma of bone. A clinical, radiographic, pathologic-anatomic, and prognostic study of 16 cases. Skeletal Radiol. 1987;16(5):364–76.

Khoddami M, Bedard YC, Bell RS, Kandel RA. Primary leiomyosarcoma of bone: report of seven cases and review of the literature. Arch Pathol Lab Med. 1996;120(7):671–75.

Peoc'h M, Vitetta F, Girard MH, Roux JJ, Plaweski S, Barnoud R, et al. Primary bone leiomyosarcoma. Anatomo-clinical case with immunohistochem istry study and review of the literature. Arch Anat Cytol Pathol. 1997;45(1):28–36.

Young MP, Freemont AJ. Primary leiomyosarcoma of bone. Histopathology. 1991;19(3):257–62.

Lymphoma of Bone

Bhagavathi S, Fu K. Primary bone lymphoma. Arch Pathol Lab Med. 2009;133(11):1868–71.

Gill P, Wenger DE, Inwards DJ. Primary lymphomas of bone. Clin Lymphoma Myeloma. 2005;6(2):140–42.

Kitsoulis P, Vlychou M, Papoudou-Bai A, Karatzias G, Charchanti A, Agnantis NJ, et al. Primary lymphomas of bone. Anticancer Res. 2006a;26((1A)):325–37.

O'Neill J, Finlay K, Jurriaans E, Friedman L. Radiological manifestations of skeletal lymphoma. Curr Probl Diagn Radiol. 2009;38(5):228–36.

Ostrowski ML, Inwards CY, Strickler JG, Witzig TE, Wenger DE, Unni KK. Osseous Hodgkin disease. Cancer. 1999;85(5):1166–78.

Pettit CK, Zukerberg LR, Gray MH, Ferry JA, Rosenberg AE, Harmon DC, et al. Primary lymphoma of bone. A B-cell neoplasm with a high frequency of multilobated cells. Am J Surg Pathol. 1990;14(4):329–34.

Malignant Fibrous Histiocytoma of Bone

Capanna R, Bertoni F, Bacchini P, Bacci G, Guerra A, Campanacci M. Malignant fibrous histiocytoma of bone. The experience at the Rizzoli Institute: report of 90 cases. Cancer. 1984;54(1):177–87.

Huvos AG, Heilweil M, Bretsky SS. The pathology of malignant fibrous histiocytoma of bone. A study of 130 patients. Am J Surg Pathol. 1985;9(12):853–71.

Little DG, McCarthy SW. Malignant fibrous histiocytoma of bone: the experience of the New South Wales Bone Tumour Registry. Aust N Z J Surg. 1993;63(5):346–51.

McCarthy EF, Matsuno T, Dorfman HD. Malignant fibrous histiocytoma of bone: a study of 35 cases. Hum Pathol. 1979;10(1):57–70.

MaNishida J, Sim FH, Wenger DE, Unni KK. Malignant fibrous histiocytoma of bone. A clinicopathologic study of 81 patients. Cancer. 1997;79(3):482–93l.

Papagelopoulos PJ, Galanis EC, Sim FH, Unni KK. Clinicopathologic features, diagnosis, and treatment of malignant fibrous histiocytoma of bone. Orthopedics. 2000;23(1):59–65. quiz 66–7.

Metastasis

Berrettoni BA, Carter JR. Mechanisms of cancer metastasis to bone. J Bone Joint Surg Am. 1986;68(2):308–12.

Bubendorf L, Schöpfer A, Wagner U, Sauter G, Moch H, Willi N, et al. Metastatic patterns of prostate cancer: an autopsy study of 1, 589 patients. Hum Pathol. 2000;31(5):578–83.

Clezardin P, Teti A. Bone metastasis: pathogenesis and therapeutic implications. Clin Exp Metastasis. 2007;24(8):599–608.

Koyama T, Hasebe T, Tsuda H, Hirohashi S, Sasaki S, Fukutomi T, et al. Histological factors associated with initial bone metastasis of invasive ductal carcinoma of the breast. Jpn J Cancer Res. 1999;90(3):294–300.

Roudier MP, Morrissey C, True LD, Higano CS, Vessella RL, Ott SM. Histopatho logical assessment of prostate cancer bone osteoblastic metastases. J Urol. 2008;180(3):1154–60.

Rougraff BT, Kneisl JS, Simon MA. Skeletal metastases of unknown origin. A prospective study of a diagnostic strategy. J Bone Joint Surg Am. 1993;75(9):1276–81.

Rubin P, Brasacchio R, Katz A. Solitary metastases: illusion versus reality. Semin Radiat Oncol. 2006;16(2):120–30.

Myeloma/Plasmacytoma

Edwards CM, Zhuang J, Mundy GR. The pathogenesis of the bone disease of multiple myeloma. Bone. 2008;42(6):1007–13.

Frassica FJ, Beabout JW, Unni KK, Sim FH. Myeloma of bone. Orthopedics. 1985;8(9):1184–86.

Knobel D, Zouhair A, Tsang RW, Poortmans P, Belkacémi Y, Bolla M, et al. Prognostic factors in solitary plasmacytoma of the bone: a multicenter Rare Cancer Network study. BMC Cancer. 2006;6:118.

Meis JM, Butler JJ, Osborne BM, Ordóñez NG. Solitary plasmacytomas of bone and extramedullary plasmacytomas. A clinicopathologic and immunohistochemical study. Cancer. 1987;59(8):1475–85.

Pambuccian SE, Horyd ID, Cawte T, Huvos AG. Amyloidoma of bone, a plasma cell/plasmacytoid neoplasm. Report of three cases and review of the literature. Am J Surg Pathol. 1997;21(2):179–86.

Roodman GD. Pathogenesis of myeloma bone disease. Leukemia. 2009;23(3):435–41.

Shaheen SP, Talwalkar SS, Medeiros LJ. Multiple myeloma and immunosecretory disorders: an update. Adv Anat Pathol. 2008;15(4):196–210.

Non-ossifying Fibroma/Metapheal Fibrous Defect

Bullough PG, Walley J. Fibrous cortical defect and non-ossifying fibroma. Postgrad Med J. 1965;41(481):672–76.

Campbell CJ, Harkess J. Fibrous metaphyseal defect of bone. Surg Gynecol Obstet. 1957;104(3):329–36.

Hau MA, Fox EJ, Cates JM, Brigman BE, Mankin HJ. Jaffe-Campanacci syndrome. A case report and review of the literature. J Bone Joint Surg Am. 2002;84-A(4):634–38.

Mankin HJ, Trahan CA, Fondren G, Mankin CJ. Non-ossifying fibroma, fibrous cortical defect and Jaffe-Campanacci syndrome: a biologic and clinical review. Chir Organi Mov. 2009;93(1):1–7.

Osteoblastoma

Baker AC, Rezeanu L, Klein MJ, Pitt MJ, Buecker P, Hersh JH, et al. Aggressive osteoblastoma: a case report involving a unique chromosomal aberration. Int J Surg Pathol. 2010;18(3):219–24.

Berry M, Mankin H, Gebhardt M, Rosenberg A, Hornicek F. Osteoblastoma: a 30-year study of 99 cases. J Surg Oncol. 2008;98(3):179–83.

Della Rocca C, Huvos AG. Osteoblastoma: varied histological presentations with a benign clinical course. An analysis of 55 cases. Am J Surg Pathol. 1996;20(7):841–50.

McLeod RA, Dahlin DC, Beabout JW. The spectrum of osteoblastoma. AJR Am J Roentgenol. 1976;126(2):321–25.

Papagelopoulos PJ, Galanis EC, Sim FH, Unni KK. Clinicopathologic features, diagnosis, and treatment of osteoblastoma. Orthopedics. 1999;22(2):244–47.

Ruggieri P, McLeod RA, Unni KK, Sim FH. Osteoblastoma. Orthopedics. 1996;19(7):621–24.

Zon Filippi R, Swee RG, Krishnan Unni K. Epithelioid multinodular osteoblastoma: a clinicopathologic analysis of 26 cases. Am J Surg Pathol. 2007;31(8):1265–68.

Osteochondroma

Bovée JV. Multiple osteochondromas. Orphanet J Rare Dis. 2008;3:3.

Kitsoulis P, Galani V, Stefanaki K, Paraskevas G, Karatzias G, Agnantis NJ, et al. Osteochondromas: review of the clinical, radiological and pathological features. In Vivo. 2008;22(5):633–46.

Porter DE, Simpson AH. The neoplastic pathogenesis of solitary and multiple osteochondromas. J Pathol. 1999;188(2):119–25.

Osteoid Osteoma

Gitelis S, Schajowicz F. Osteoid osteoma and osteoblastoma. Orthop Clin North Am. 1989;20(3):313–25.

Greenspan A. Benign bone-forming lesions: osteoma, osteoid osteoma, and osteoblastoma. Clinical, imaging, pathologic, and differential considerations. Skeletal Radiol. 1993;22(7):485–500.

Jaffe HL. Osteoid-osteoma. Proc R Soc Med. 1953;46(12):1007–12.

Kitsoulis P, Mantellos G, Vlychou M. Osteoid osteoma. Acta Orthop Belg. 2006b;72(2):119–25.

O'Connell JX, Nanthakumar SS, Nielsen GP, Rosenberg AE. Osteoid osteoma: the uniquely innervated bone tumor. Mod Pathol. 1998;11(2):175–80.

Osteosarcoma

Antonescu CR, Huvos AG. Low-grade osteogenic sarcoma arising in medullary and surface osseous locations. Am J Clin Pathol. 2000;114(Suppl):S90–S103.

Ayala AG, Ro JY, Papadopoulos NK, Raymond AK, Edeiken J. Small cell osteosarcoma. Cancer Treat Res. 1993;62:139–49.

Huvos AG, Rosen G, Bretsky SS, Butler A. Telangiectatic osteogenic sarcoma: a clinicopathologic study of 124 patients. Cancer. 1982;49(8):1679–89.

Klein MJ, Siegal GP. Osteosarcoma: anatomic and histologic variants. Am J Clin Pathol. 2006;125(4):555–81.

Nakajima H, Sim FH, Bond JR, Unni KK. Small cell osteosarcoma of bone. Review of 72 cases. Cancer. 1997;79(11):2095–106.

Rosen G, Caparros B, Huvos AG, Kosloff C, Nirenberg A, Cacavio A, et al. Preoperative chemotherapy for osteogenic sarcoma: selection of postoperative adjuvant chemotherapy based on the response of the primary tumor to preoperative chemotherapy. Cancer. 1982;49(6):1221–30.

Sheth DS, Yasko AW, Raymond AK, Ayala AG, Carrasco CH, Benjamin RS, et al. Conventional and dedifferentiated parosteal osteosarcoma. Diagnosis, treatment, and outcome. Cancer. 1996;78(10):2136–45.

Unni KK, Dahlin DC. Osteosarcoma: pathology and classification. Semin Roentgenol. 1989;24(3):143–52.

Unni KK, Dahlin DC, Beabout JW. Periosteal osteogenic sarcoma. Cancer. 1976b;37(5):2476–85.

Unni KK, Dahlin DC, Beabout JW, Ivins JC. Parosteal osteogenic sarcoma. Cancer. 1976c;37(5):2466–75.

Unni KK, Dahlin DC, McLeod RA, Pritchard DJ. Intraosseous well-differentiated osteosarcoma. Cancer. 1977;40(3):1337–47.

Unicameral/Solitary Bone Cyst

Boseker EH, Bickel WH, Dahlin DC. A clinicopathologic study of simple unicameral bone cysts. Surg Gynecol Obstet. 1968;127(3):550–60.

Capanna R, Campanacci DA, Manfrini M. Unicameral and aneurysmal bone cysts. Orthop Clin North Am. 1996;27(3):605–14.

Harnet JC, Lombardi T, Klewansky P, Rieger J, Tempe MH, Clavert JM. Solitary bone cyst of the jaws: a review of the etiopathogenic hypotheses. J Oral Maxillofac Surg. 2008;66(11):2345–48.

Index